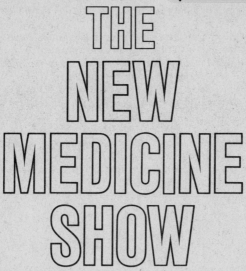

THE NEW MEDICINE SHOW

Consumers Union's Practical Guide to Some Everyday Health Problems and Health Products

By the Editors of

CONSUMER REPORTS BOOKS

A PORTION OF THIS BOOK IS MADE WITH
RECYCLED PAPER.

CONSUMERS UNION
Mount Vernon, New York

Library of Congress Cataloging-in-Publication Data
The new medicine show : Consumers Union's practical guide to some everyday health problems and health products / by the editors of Consumer Reports Books.—6th ed.

p.   cm.

Rev. ed. of: The medicine show. 5th ed. 1980.
Includes indexes.
ISBN 0-89043-237-6

1. Medicine, Popular.   2. Quacks and quackery.   3. Health products.   4. Consumer education.   I. Consumers Union of United States.   II. Consumer Reports Books.   III. Medicine show.
RC81.N525   1988

613—dc 19

88-13776
CIP

First published 1961
Second edition 1963
Third edition 1971
Fourth edition 1974; updated September 1976
Fifth edition 1980; updated January 1983
Sixth edition 1989
Design by Tamara O'Bradovich
Manufactured in the United States of America

CONTENTS

PREFACE

This sixth edition of *The Medicine Show,* like the earlier ones, is based on articles originally published in the pages of *Consumer Reports,* the monthly magazine of Consumers Union. The material in this book has been extensively rewritten, updated, and expanded, with the assistance of Consumers Union's medical and dental consultants.

A number of publications were consulted in the preparation of *The New Medicine Show.* Basic sources, frequently cited in this edition, include *The Pharmacological Basis of Therapeutics,* 7th edition (Macmillan), a pharmacology, toxicology, and therapeutics text for physicians and medical students, edited by Louis S. Goodman, M.D., and Alfred Gilman, Ph.D.; *AMA Drug Evaluations,* 6th edition (Department of Drugs, American Medical Association); *Handbook of Nonprescription Drugs,* 8th edition (American Pharmaceutical Association); and *The Medical Letter,* a nonprofit periodical for medical professionals containing drug evaluations in terms of effectiveness, safety, and possible alternatives. Other major references include the published reports of the FDA's OTC Drug Review Program (discussed in the Introduction).

ACKNOWLEDGMENTS

*The editors of Consumer Reports Books
wish to give special thanks
to the following people for the contributions
and reviews they provided:*
Joseph R. Botta
Michael Leff
Jonathan Leff
Marvin M. Lipman, M.D.
Irwin D. Mandel, D.D.S.

Introduction

Many "everyday health problems" are more annoying than dangerous, more a bother than a threat. Left to their own devices, most people would be quite capable of coping with such problems. But people are not left alone. Indeed, they are all but overwhelmed by "news" stories of miraculous medical discoveries, by testimonials—some gratuitous, some paid—from satisfied users, by broadcast commercials, print advertisements, and label claims on thousands of products filling the shelves of drugstores and supermarkets. Not only is their peace disturbed, often their money is wasted. And sometimes their health is threatened.

It is truly a medicine show. No one questions the energy, ingenuity, or skill of its promoters. Nor are they all crude hawkers of snake oil; some of the sales pitches are positively low-keyed. What thoughtful consumers should challenge is the extent to which the hucksters succeed in becoming the medical educators of the buyers. Virtually all promoters of health products "educate" the public in the same way: Since selling is their prime purpose, they state no more than what is in their interest. All too often it is in their interest to exploit popular concern about a health problem, real or imagined—for which their product is the ultimate and only true remedy.

Huckstering should not be confused with education, particularly education on matters of health and medicine. Yet many people do confuse the two. A few years ago, the U.S. Food and Drug Administration (FDA) reported the results of a study of American health practices and opinions. Those surveyed were presented with the statement that advertisements about medications and health aids "must be true or they wouldn't be allowed to say them." Of those surveyed, 38 percent—representing 50 million Americans 18 and over—agreed with the statement.

Reliable information on health and medicine is needed, and Consumers Union looks to the time when responsible drug advertising will help better meet that need. Meanwhile, this book offers consumers "a restorative of balance and perspective, an antidote to excesses, and a purgative for much nonsense"—as stated in 1961 in the first edition of *The Medicine Show*. Completely revised and brought up to date, this latest edition

1

is intended to help consumers better understand the differences between genuine advances in health and medicine and the frequently distorted claims of the sellers.

Old familiar "miracles" of drug advertising still burst upon the scene, only to fade away and be followed by new ones. Regulations catch up with deceptions. New fads replace old ones. Fresh claims are cranked out to beguile the consumer.

But many consumers still refuse to be sold by the hucksters' medicine show. Like CU, they question the propriety and the quality of drug advertising as a source of information about health and medicine. This new edition of *The Medicine Show,* like the earlier ones, is addressed not only to these skeptics and truth seekers, but also to those who may still be susceptible to the blandishments of the hucksters.

The New Medicine Show seeks to help consumers make better choices—when choices are available—in many areas of health and medicine. In addition to the familiar world of over-the-counter (OTC) drugs, the book offers some insights into the puzzling world of prescription drugs, where the pharmaceutical company provides, the physician prescribes, the pharmacist fulfills, and the patient—the consumer—pays.

The thinking of many consultants to Consumers Union—physicians and other health professionals—is represented here, and health professionals should find the book a useful adjunct to their efforts to give their patients sound guidance in medical matters. But *The New Medicine Show* is not primarily for health professionals, nor even for patients. It is above all for consumers who want a source of health information significantly more reliable than the next television commercial.

OTC DRUGS AND THE FDA'S REVIEW PROGRAM

The OTC drug marketplace—the main attraction at the medicine show— is slowly changing, due to an ambitious undertaking by the FDA.

The 1938 U.S. Food, Drug and Cosmetic Act required that all drugs introduced after that date must be safe for human use. Until a 1951 amendment, the distinction between prescription and nonprescription drugs remained blurred. The amendment mandated prescriptions for all drugs that cannot be used safely without medical supervision—such as those that are habit-forming, toxic, potentially harmful, or new and unproven. Drugs that were none of those things could still be sold over the counter. In 1962, further amendments required that all drugs be shown to be effective for their intended uses. Most of the OTC drugs approved for safety since 1938 had never been proved effective.

In 1972 the FDA inaugurated an extensive OTC Drug Review Program to ensure that drugs are both safe *and* effective for their intended purposes. The review program involves advisory panels of medical and scientific authorities, with an industry and a consumer representative assigned to each panel. The panels were charged by the FDA with the responsibility of reviewing and evaluating more than 700 active ingredients used in approximately 300,000 nonprescription drug products. These ingredients were divided into about 80 therapeutic categories (such as cough and cold medications, antacids, skin protectants, and so on), each of which was assigned to one of 17 advisory panels. Also included for review by the panels were the labeling claims and other statements relevant to the drugs, such as warnings and directions for use.

Once its review is completed, a panel's recommendations—which are not binding on the FDA—are published in the *Federal Register* in order to elicit consumer and industry comment. After public comments have been evaluated, the FDA then publishes a tentative final monograph in the *Federal Register* to invite public response once again. Evaluation of the second series of public comments leads eventually to the final monograph, which has the effect of law.

The panel review stage of the program took nearly a decade. Panel recommendations, tentative monographs, and final monographs have followed, and the process continues even now. As of August 1988, all panels had submitted their recommendations, and 21 of the recommendations had been published in final form.

Although the final regulations on all OTC drug categories are probably several years away, ingredients that were not shown to be both safe and effective have already been dropped from many OTC formulations, and certain remedies have disappeared altogether. Some products have been reformulated or are in the process of being reformulated as panel recommendations become known. Eventually, many more products will have to be reformulated or withdrawn from the market. However, there are still many OTC remedies currently on the market that do not meet the FDA review panels' recommended guidelines.

In searching for an OTC remedy, then, bear in mind that brand-name identity is no substitute for careful reading of the list of ingredients. That's especially necessary now, since manufacturers are in the process of changing some products to meet the established or anticipated final monograph regulations. A familiar product today may have entirely different ingredients tomorrow.

Most drugs contain large amounts of "pharmaceutical manufacturing necessities," otherwise known as inactive ingredients. They include preservatives, coating agents, colors, flavors, sweeteners, buffers, lubricants, solvents, and other additives. Under the law, the FDA can require only that active ingredients be listed on an OTC drug's label. However, one or more of the inactive ingredients might cause problems for certain people—those who are allergic, for example. In the case of cosmetics, *all* the ingredients are inactive, yet by law they must be listed on cosmetic labeling. Consumers Union's medical consultants think the same should be required of all OTC drugs as well. Many manufacturers list toll-free "800" numbers on their packaging. These information lines may be able to reveal any hidden inactive ingredients that might trouble you.

The New Medicine Show includes frequent references to products by brand name, often in discussions of specific products. In general discussions, brand names—particularly of drugs, both prescription and OTC—are mentioned as examples and for ease of identification. For example, a widely prescribed anticoagulant is referred to in the text as "warfarin (Athrombin-K, Coumadin, Panwarfin)"; *warfarin* is the drug's generic name and in parentheses are the names of some brands of warfarin. Such references are not intended as endorsements or as a comprehensive listing of all brands available. For identification purposes the brand names of prescription drugs are capitalized while brand names of OTC drugs are capitalized and italicized.

The New Medicine Show includes a glossary of select words and phrases related to health and medicine. We urge readers to use the glossary for a better understanding not only of this book but of medical language that may be encountered elsewhere.

I

REMEDIES
for
COMMON
COMPLAINTS

1

Competing Pain Relievers: Aspirin, Acetaminophen, and Ibuprofen

Few things seem to appeal to drug companies more than the opportunity to sell you a nonprescription pain reliever. Eager to share in this lucrative market, they offer an oriental bazaar of choices.

You may find more than 100 different analgesic products competing for space on the shelves at your local drugstore or supermarket. There are "original" formulas, "new" formulas, and "advanced" formulas. There are tablets, capsules, "caplets," liquids, and gum. They come in "regular" strength, "extra" strength, and, presumably for those in real agony, "maximum" strength. And the price of the products may vary dramatically, by tenfold or more.

All this apparent variety ends, though, when you examine the ingredients. Inside each package, there is usually only one of three common analgesics: aspirin, acetaminophen, or ibuprofen.

The U.S. Food and Drug Administration (FDA) considers all three effective for the same minor aches and pains. Each can reduce fever and relieve headache, muscle aches, menstrual pain, toothache, and similar discomfort—although they differ somewhat in their effectiveness against certain of these symptoms. For the vast majority of people, occasional use of any of the three analgesics is quite safe. However, each of them can cause unpleasant or serious side effects in certain individuals.

ASPIRIN: THE LEADER

Ever since it was first marketed at the turn of the century, aspirin has reigned as the nation's leading analgesic. And it has remained popular because it works.

7

Two 325-milligram tablets can relieve mild-to-moderate pain and reduce fever. Its action against inflammation also makes aspirin a first-line drug in treating arthritis, although much higher doses are required for this anti-inflammatory effect.

Side Effects

One well-publicized side effect of aspirin is its interference with the function of platelets, blood cells that enable blood to clot. This can be either an added benefit or a dangerous drawback, depending on the user. Clinical studies show that small doses of aspirin apparently reduce the risk of blood clots that can lead to stroke and heart attack. However, because of this blood-"thinning" side effect, people with bleeding tendencies or patients taking anticoagulants must avoid using aspirin. For many individuals, in fact, the known risks of taking aspirin will outweigh its potential benefit against cardiovascular disease.

Recently, initial results from a controlled five-year study of 22,000 healthy male U.S. physicians aged 40 to 84 years were released. According to the report, one 325-milligram aspirin tablet taken every other day reduced the incidence of heart attack in the subject population by 47 percent. However, the participants represented a highly selected population: male physicians with no history of heart attack or stroke, and with *no contraindications* to the use of aspirin. For the general population, it's not yet certain who stands to benefit from such therapy. Ethical concerns about doing additional studies may prompt doctors to rely on results already in hand. Because the risks are as real as the potential rewards, any decision to undertake a regular regimen of aspirin therapy should be made in consultation with a physician.

Other studies have shown a benefit from aspirin therapy (usually one 325-milligram tablet a day) in patients with a history of cardiovascular disease. In men, such intervention lowers the risk of stroke and transient ischemic attacks (brief episodes of strokelike symptoms). It also helps prevent heart attacks in men with unstable angina (chest pains that have recently worsened). And in both men and women who survive an initial heart attack, aspirin appears to reduce the risk of a subsequent attack.

Another common side effect of aspirin, but one that has no redeeming value, is its tendency to irritate the stomach. Between 2 percent and 10 percent of all those who use aspirin—even only occasionally—experience mild stomach upset or nausea. With occasional usage, serious gastrointestinal effects are uncommon; however, heavy chronic users, such as those with arthritis, face an increased risk of severe stomach bleeding from ulceration and inflammation. Anyone with ulcers or other stomach problems should avoid taking aspirin, except under the supervision of a physician. Heavy chronic usage may also lead to iron-deficiency anemia, caused by the cumulative loss, over a long period of time, of small amounts of blood—too small to be visible—in the stool.

Buffered aspirin, which includes small amounts of antacid, has been promoted as "faster" and "gentler" than plain aspirin—but don't count on it. Clinical studies comparing plain and buffered aspirin for speed of pain relief found no difference. And in other studies, researchers examined the stomach linings of people taking plain and buffered aspirin and found no difference in damage.

Enteric-coated aspirin, on the other hand, does cause less stomach irritation. The tablets have a special coating that prevents them from dissolving until they reach the small intestine. While such slow-dissolving tablets don't give prompt relief, they can benefit those who take high daily doses.

A small percentage of individuals, often those with severe asthma or chronic hives, are aspirin-sensitive and must avoid the drug altogether.

Pregnant women should also forgo aspirin (as well as most other drugs—see Chapter 22, "Drugs in Pregnancy"), especially during the last three months of pregnancy. At that stage, aspirin may prolong pregnancy and labor and increase the possibility of maternal bleeding, stillbirth, and infant mortality.

Children who have, or are recovering from, flu or chicken pox should never be given aspirin. Studies indicate that aspirin given to children with these illnesses may cause Reye's syndrome, a rare but often fatal disorder. Early in 1986, the FDA required that all aspirin-containing products bear labels warning about this risk. Acetaminophen is an acceptable substitute.

Aspirin in Chewing Gum

We do not recommend aspirin-containing chewing gum. *Aspergum* has been advertised "for minor sore throat pain"—yet aspirin has no topical anesthetic or analgesic action. Any benefit derived from this type of preparation comes from its absorption into the bloodstream from the intestinal tract once the saliva/aspirin mixture is swallowed. And even then, while it may help relieve general discomfort that often accompanies a sore throat, it won't relieve the sore throat itself, which is one of the types of pain for which relief is difficult to achieve. Gargling with aspirin dissolved in water should be avoided because of the possible irritating effect of aspirin particles on the gums and mucosal lining of the throat and mouth. Instead, stick with the traditional sore throat remedy: frequent gargling with warm salt water (see page 29).

What about *Aspergum*'s utility as a way to ingest aspirin for other, more appropriate types of pain? One piece of *Aspergum* contains only about 70 percent of the aspirin in the usual 325-milligram tablet. It would be more effective and much cheaper to swallow an aspirin tablet—and then have a piece of sugarless gum, if you like. One further caution: An FDA advisory panel on internal analgesics has warned against the use of chewable aspirin and aspirin-containing gum during the week following any oral surgery, including tonsillectomy, to avoid irritating oral tissues.

ACETAMINOPHEN: CLOSING FAST

While many people may not know the word *acetaminophen,* almost everyone has heard of *Tylenol.* Sold by McNeil Laboratories, a division of Johnson & Johnson, the *Tylenol* brand of acetaminophen may rank among America's foremost marketing successes. In 1987, the various versions of *Tylenol* enjoyed a higher sales volume than all the major brands of aspirin products combined.

That's less a tribute to the superiority of acetaminophen than to the power of advertising. Many people seem unaware that other choices exist, which may explain the hefty price *Tylenol* commands; it generally costs more than other brands of acetaminophen, such as *Anacin-3, Datril,* and *Panadol,* and often much more than generic versions. According to pharmacology experts, acetaminophen is a drug that's "hard to ruin" when compounding the active ingredient into pills. So competing brands of acetaminophen should work just as well as *Tylenol.* And they do.

Acetaminophen shares aspirin's ability to relieve mild-to-moderate pain and to reduce fever, but it lacks aspirin's anti-inflammatory effect. Although acetaminophen can help to relieve pain *caused* by inflammation, it can't relieve this type of pain as effectively because it can't reduce the underlying inflammation itself.

Acetaminophen may be a safe alternative for those who can't take aspirin for some reason, but its most common advantage is that it tends to be less irritating to the stomach.

Side Effects

While acetaminophen causes few side effects of any kind at normal doses, it's not totally nonirritating, despite commercials to the contrary. Johnson & Johnson, which has touted *Tylenol*'s "gentleness" in TV ads, was more candid in a brochure for health professionals, acknowledging that *Tylenol* may sometimes cause stomach upset at recommended doses.

One group of people—active alcoholics—should avoid acetaminophen. Their alcohol intake makes them susceptible to liver damage from acetaminophen, even with moderate doses of the drug. In contrast to the relative ease of treating aspirin poisoning, overdosage with acetaminophen is difficult to treat and often fatal.

IBUPROFEN: THE NEWCOMER

The FDA created front-page news in 1984 when it approved the marketing of two new pain relievers, *Advil* and *Nuprin.* Both products contained ibuprofen as their active ingredient. Ibuprofen was the first new over-the-counter (OTC) analgesic since 1955, when acetaminophen was introduced.

Analysts predicted instant success for ibuprofen. After all, a prescription-strength version, Motrin, was a proven winner; on the market since 1974, it was being widely prescribed for arthritis and menstrual pain. But after two years *Advil* and *Nuprin* had captured only 15 percent of the OTC analgesic market. Then a bevy of new brands—*Haltran, Medipren, Trendar Ibuprofen, Ibuprin, Midol 200,* and others—entered the competition when exclusive marketing rights for *Advil* and *Nuprin* expired in 1986. Within a year, ibuprofen had garnered 20 percent of the market. Some analysts predict its share will continue to increase until it accounts for as much as one-third of all OTC analgesic sales.

Aspirin and ibuprofen seem to work the same way in the body. Both drugs inhibit the production of prostaglandins, hormonelike chemicals involved in causing pain and inflammation.

Side Effects

Ironically, the inhibition of prostaglandin production also plays a role in stomach upset, the most common side effect of both aspirin and ibuprofen. Prostaglandins exert a protective effect on the stomach lining. By inhibiting this action, those drugs increase the chances of stomach upset. Stomach upset occurs less often with ibuprofen, however, because aspirin has an added direct irritating effect on the stomach lining. On a "stomach-upset scale," ibuprofen stands somewhere between aspirin (more irritating) and acetaminophen (less irritating).

Concerns over ibuprofen's safety were raised when the FDA approved the drug for OTC sale. Some physicians pointed out that nonprescription ibuprofen could pose serious health risks of possible kidney damage for certain people.

After OTC ibuprofen had been on the market for two years, CU asked the FDA for an update on adverse effects. We were told by agency spokesman William Grigg that "it does not appear that over-the-counter ibuprofen has caused either frequent or serious effects" of any kind. Grigg did say, however, that the FDA had reports of 14 cases of kidney problems among people who were taking OTC ibuprofen.

THE SHOTGUN APPROACH

People in pain are often persuaded by the ads to buy remedies containing several ingredients—apparently on the theory that if there are enough of them, at least one might work. Such "shotgun" recipes may include combinations of aspirin, acetaminophen, salicylamide (chemically related to aspirin, but different enough to be considered ineffective by the FDA, and now nearly obsolete), caffeine, and various antacids.

The so-called buffering effect of antacids in aspirin products has already been questioned. As for caffeine, the authoritative handbook

AMA Drug Evaluations reports conflicting findings. "Although results of some studies have suggested that caffeine may increase the analgesic effect of aspirin or acetaminophen, others have not substantiated such enhancement. Thus," the text concludes, "mixtures of analgesic-antipyretic drugs with or without caffeine have not been proved to be superior to optimal doses of the individual components."

In fact, CU knows of no conclusive proof that *any* multiple-drug analgesic combination is superior—milligram for milligram—to a single-ingredient product. What's more, a combination product exposes an individual to the allergic potential of two or more ingredients. In its *Handbook of Nonprescription Drugs,* the American Pharmaceutical Association notes: "Few well-controlled studies support the enhanced efficacy of such combinations." We recommend that you stick to the single drug most appropriate to your needs and restrictions.

Compared to the stupefying variety of aspirin and acetaminophen brands, ibuprofen has seemed the soul of simplicity. There are as yet no buffers or other added ingredients, no "extra-" or "maximum-strength" formulas. So far, every single brand of ibuprofen, including generic versions, consists of a tablet (or caplet) containing 200 milligrams of the drug. (However, ibuprofen has been approved as a substitute for aspirin or acetaminophen in certain shotgun cough and cold remedies.)

Beginning with CU's first look at aspirin products in 1936, we've given consumers this basic advice: Brands with similar amounts of the same active ingredient should work equally well. That's true for all three analgesics—and especially so for the flurry of new ibuprofen brands. You won't go wrong if you buy the cheapest one.

COMPARING PAIN RELIEF

Pain and its relief are extremely subjective and difficult to measure. So it's not surprising that comparisons of pain relievers have long posed problems for researchers. In a typical clinical study, a high percentage of patients with pain—30 to 40 percent—will show marked improvement even when given a placebo. Nevertheless, some useful conclusions can be drawn from head-to-head contests that have been conducted with the three drugs.

Milligram for milligram, aspirin and acetaminophen are equally potent for relieving pain—equally fast and equally enduring. With either drug, two regular-strength 325-milligram tablets—650 milligrams total—can take care of most headaches and other minor aches and pains. A third tablet usually isn't necessary, although it may help when pain is more severe.

Ibuprofen appears to offer some pain-relief advantages over its two competitors. For one thing, studies suggest that one 200-milligram tablet provides slightly greater pain relief than 650 milligrams of either aspirin or acetaminophen. Label directions advise taking two tablets of ibuprofen if one doesn't help, and clinical studies suggest that the extra dose can make a modest difference.

There is no additional advantage in taking more than two tablets of ibuprofen—400 milligrams total—for ordinary aches and pains. Several studies have found that higher dosages don't increase the level or duration of relief for mild-to-moderate pain. However, dosages of up to 800 milligrams at a time are used in relieving arthritis pain, when consistently high blood levels of ibuprofen are required.

Ibuprofen's principal virtues involve the *types* of pain it can relieve. For example, it appears quite helpful for treating pain from "soft tissue" injuries such as strains and sprains. Ibuprofen has also done well in studies involving pain relief after dental surgery. But the main reason the FDA approved the drug for OTC sale is its effectiveness against menstrual pain.

Easing Menstrual Pain

About half of all American women of childbearing age experience menstrual discomfort, or dysmenorrhea. The symptoms—cramping and lower abdominal and back pain—generally occur during the first two days of the menstrual period. The discomfort causes 10 percent of women to lose significant time from school or work each month.

Dysmenorrhea most commonly affects teenagers and usually diminishes or disappears entirely when a woman reaches her twenties or after she gives birth. But some women continue to experience discomfort well into their thirties or beyond.

Dysmenorrhea appears to be caused by prostaglandins that the uterus produces during menstruation. Because ibuprofen dramatically decreases prostaglandin production, it can relieve the cramping and pain. Studies show that it provides complete or significant relief for 75 percent of dysmenorrhea patients.

For best results, ibuprofen should be taken at the start of the menstrual flow and continued for 24 to 48 hours. Studies show no advantage to taking ibuprofen before the period begins.

A number of brand-name products are promoted specifically for menstrual pain. Consider such specific advertising a reason to choose another product containing ibuprofen. Most products promoted for menstrual pain contain aspirin or acetaminophen rather than ibuprofen. While effective to some extent, these drugs don't work as well as ibuprofen does for this symptom.

The newest menstrual-pain products do contain ibuprofen—but cost far more than those ibuprofen brands that are not targeted exclusively for this purpose. Strictly a marketing strategy, the higher price is intended to bolster their image as "high-tech" pain relievers. The manufacturers also hope that a woman who starts out taking an ibuprofen product sold specifically for menstrual pain will stick with it if it works, rather than try something cheaper. As mentioned earlier, however, all OTC ibuprofen products offer exactly the same dose: 200 milligrams per unit. They should all be equally effective against menstrual pain.

MAKING YOUR SELECTION

For occasional relief of garden-variety aches and pains, most healthy individuals won't go wrong with any of the three analgesics.

Most people with chronic disorders can also take any one of the three drugs without harm, provided its use is occasional and limited to a day or so. For frequent or extended use, a physician should be consulted—especially if the chronic ailment also requires the daily use of a medication, such as a diuretic or insulin. If you do have a chronic disorder—regardless of whether it requires medication—the safest course is to ask your physician in advance about OTC pain relievers. This is particularly important if you have ulcers, kidney impairment, high blood pressure, liver problems, congestive heart failure, gout, or diabetes.

People in their late sixties and older should also check with their physicians about use of OTC pain relievers. Undetected kidney impairment and hypertension often affect older people; both problems can be aggravated by ibuprofen and, to a lesser extent, by aspirin.

In general, anyone who should avoid aspirin for any reason should also avoid ibuprofen—and vice versa. Both drugs work the same way and can cause similar side effects.

Although people with arthritis are the most likely customers for large amounts of aspirin or ibuprofen, they shouldn't try to diagnose or treat the disease themselves. Joint pain can arise from many disorders, including osteoarthritis, rheumatoid arthritis, gout, pseudogout, and others. Inadequate treatment can lead to irreversible joint damage, and the large doses of either drug needed for effective pain relief substantially increase the risk of side effects. Consequently, anyone with significant arthritic complaints should be under a physician's care and should ignore advertisements for OTC pain relievers.

Apart from the caveats discussed in this chapter, plain generic or store brands of aspirin are, in most instances, as good as any OTC pain reliever—and much less expensive than acetaminophen, ibuprofen, or the heavily promoted brands of aspirin. So, if you have no health reasons for avoiding aspirin, it's a reasonable first choice.

For those who cannot tolerate aspirin and who don't require anti-inflammatory action, acetaminophen is an acceptable substitute. We recommend acetaminophen specifically for people who are allergic to aspirin; have stomach disorders, kidney disease, gout, bleeding tendencies; or are taking anticoagulants, antidiabetics, or arthritis drugs other than aspirin.

For certain miseries, ibuprofen may be more effective than either aspirin or acetaminophen. It's superior to both for menstrual cramps. And it's apparently more effective for postsurgical dental pain and for soft-tissue injuries such as sprains.

To minimize stomach upset, take any analgesic with a full glass of water or other liquid. If it still upsets your stomach, switch to one of the other two drugs.

For children's doses of pain reliever, consult the label. For those under two years old, consult a physician. Children who dislike taking tablets (even crushed and disguised in some applesauce) may prefer liquid acetaminophen. Avoid orange-flavored children's aspirin or fruit-flavored acetaminophen; their tempting similarity to candy poses a real risk of fatal overdose to infants and toddlers.

Adults who have trouble swallowing pills may also prefer liquid pain relievers—although the convenience generally costs more. Ibuprofen and plain aspirin do not come in liquid form, but you can buy aspirin-containing products that are soluble in water, such as *Alka-Seltzer Effervescent Antacid and Pain Reliever.* However, this *Alka-Seltzer* product contains so much sodium bicarbonate that it should *not* be taken daily over long periods. And its sodium content is so high that it should not be used *at all* by anyone on a low-salt diet, as the current label warns.

Choline salicylate, a compound related to aspirin, does come in liquid form and is marketed under the name *Arthropan Liquid.* According to the American Pharmaceutical Association's *Handbook of Nonprescription Drugs,* choline salicylate seems to be somewhat less potent than aspirin; however, it may produce less gastrointestinal bleeding and distress.

If you are limited in your choice of an analgesic because of health reasons, price naturally becomes secondary. But when all other factors are equal, let the price decide.

2

Colds, Coughs, and Sore Throats

Beginning with the discovery of penicillin in 1928, there has been more progress toward the prevention and treatment of infectious diseases in the past sixty years than in all the rest of medical history combined. Smallpox has been eradicated, typhoid fever has become a rarity, and pneumococcal pneumonia is both curable and preventable, to name just a few successes. But no means has yet been found to eliminate the common cold. The only cures remain the body's natural defenses and the passage of time.

ANATOMY OF A COLD

A cold is primarily an infection of the membrane lining the upper respiratory tract, including the nose, the sinuses, and the throat. This delicate membrane reacts to infection by swelling and by increasing its rate of mucus formation, leading to congestion, stuffiness, and a great deal of nose blowing. When the nasal cavity is lost as a resonating chamber, a characteristic change in the cold sufferer's voice quality also occurs. The increased mucus flow usually causes a postnasal drip, which is irritating and contributes to the familiar "scratchy" throat and cough.

The sinuses, which normally empty into the nasal cavity, may become blocked by excessive swelling of the membranes. The increase in sinus pressure that results may cause a "sinus headache." In similar fashion, swelling in the back of the throat can block the Eustachian tubes—the two narrow canals that extend from the throat to the ears. This blockage can cause accumulation of fluid and pressure in the middle ear, which may be painful. Less commonly, an unpleasant spinning sensation—vertigo—may result, accompanied at times by nausea and vomiting.

A cold is self-limiting, usually lasting about one to two weeks. At any time during the course of a cold, bacteria (such as staphylococci, streptococci, or pneumococci) can be secondary invaders, bringing on painful infections of the sinuses and ears. However, the old admonition that a cold will turn into pneumonia if you don't take care is hardly ever true. Pneumonia and most other infections of the lower respiratory tract begin in the bronchi and the lungs rather than in the upper respiratory tract.

Most people stay home from work or school because of generalized symptoms—muscle aches, weakness, and fatigue. The extent of these symptoms varies from person to person, and from cold to cold. Although mild elevation of temperature can occur with the common cold, an oral temperature above 101°F is usually a sign of a more serious viral or bacterial infection. If fever above 101°F persists beyond two days, medical advice should be sought.

HOW COLDS ARE TRANSMITTED

Scientists believe that the "common cold" is actually some 200 different infections caused by 200 different viruses. Each infection may result in lifetime immunity, so each cold endured means one less virus to worry about. Indeed, people generally get fewer colds as they get older. Immunity is partly responsible, but another factor—less contact with children as we age—may be even more important.

Children's noses have been called "the chief reservoirs of infectious rhinoviruses," the class of viruses responsible for 30 to 50 percent of all colds. Preschoolers have the most colds—from 6 to 10 a year—and young parents often catch them from their children.

Now just as sixty years ago—regardless of any physical measure, diet, or drug—Americans will suffer an average of two to three colds a year. U.S. Public Health Service studies show that during the winter 50 percent of the population will experience at least one common cold; the figure drops to 20 percent during the summer.

Why the seasonal variation? Contrary to popular belief, studies involving volunteers exposed to the elements show that cold, wetness, and drafts don't increase the chances of catching a cold. There is no evidence that the common cold ever occurs by such "spontaneous generation"; that is, a cold cannot arise without an infecting organism. Moreover, studies have shown that chilling does not predispose one to infection by a cold virus—although excessively low humidity might. The increased incidence of colds in winter merely reflects the fact that people spend more time crowded together indoors, thereby making it easier for viruses to spread from person to person. In fact, one is far less likely to catch a cold during exposure to the elements than at a fireside gathering with a convivial group of snifflers and sneezers.

Experts disagree on how colds are transmitted. Some say through the air—in the mist created by a sneeze, for example. But evidence favors direct contact as the main route, such as shaking hands with a cold sufferer who has just blown his or her nose.

It's probably easier to catch a cold by shaking hands than by kissing. Cold viruses are present in very low amounts in saliva. Studies of kissing couples—one with a cold, one without—found that osculation seldom led to inoculation.

Resistance seems to vary greatly among individuals, so that not everyone exposed to a common source of infection becomes ill. Moreover, the natural factors—whatever they are—that contribute to resistance in an individual may be operative at one time and not another. Thus it is not uncommon for some unlucky person to have a "bad year," suffering from as many as five or six colds, and then to remain virtually cold-free during the next year or two.

Some preventive measures may help break the chain of infection. Use tissues rather than handkerchiefs; cold viruses don't survive as long on tissues. Wash your hands frequently when someone in your house has a cold. And try to keep your fingers away from your nose and eyes.

COLD REMEDIES

Cold remedies of today come no closer to curing colds or shortening their duration than did folk treatments thousands of years ago. Nevertheless, today's remedies can relieve some of the vexing symptoms. That's a big improvement since the early 1970s, when leading brands such as *Contac, Dristan,* and *NyQuil* contained decongestants in doses too paltry to do any good. Now they and other cold remedies have been beefed up. In fact, the potency of over-the-counter (OTC) cold products rivals anything requiring a prescription.

But two major flaws persist. Today most cold products are still "shotgun" remedies, loaded with up to seven different drugs. Users often waste money on unnecessary drugs that can cause unwanted side effects. In addition, one of the main drugs in these shotgun cold remedies—the antihistamine—is a dud.

Antihistamines: Blank Ammunition Antihistamines are useful for hay fever and similar allergies. Pollen and other allergens can cause cells in the nose to release histamine, a chemical that inflames nasal tissue and causes runny nose, congestion, and sneezing. An antihistamine minimizes these allergy symptoms by blocking the action of histamine.

Histamine plays no demonstrable role in colds, however. So any action of antihistamine on colds arises from the drug's side effects. In addition to inducing drowsiness, antihistamines cause some drying of nasal secretions. But that effect is so slight as to be almost undetectable.

In 1972 the U.S. Food and Drug Administration (FDA) appointed a panel of experts to evaluate the ingredients in cold remedies. The panel reported in 1976 that there was insufficient evidence to show that antihistamines worked against colds. It relegated the drugs to "Category 3" status, an official designation indicating that they lacked proof of efficacy.

Subsequently, however, studies sponsored by Schering Corporation, the maker of several cold remedies, persuaded the FDA to overrule its panel. The Schering studies found that chlorpheniramine maleate, a commonly used antihistamine, modestly outperformed a placebo in relieving two cold symptoms—runny nose and sneezing. In a leap of faith, the FDA concluded that nine other antihistamines should also work against those symptoms.

The FDA's conclusions proved premature. In late 1987, a symposium of specialists in ear, nose, and throat diseases appraised the value of antihistamines in treating colds. Three researchers presented new results from controlled clinical studies. In contrast to the Schering studies, which relied solely on subjective appraisals of relief, these studies also assessed drug effects with sophisticated instruments that measured changes in nasal airflow, middle-ear pressure, and other objective parameters.

None of the studies found antihistamines significantly more effective than a placebo in relieving cold symptoms. The symposium's consensus statement summarized the findings: "The data appear to be conclusive that antihistamines do not have a place in the management of upper respiratory infection, though they continue to be useful for allergy."

We believe that the FDA should ban antihistamines from cold remedies. They don't work, and the drowsiness they cause can be hazardous for people who must operate machinery or drive—or a nuisance for anyone just trying to stay alert.

Shotgun Remedies: Too Much and Too Little   Few drugstore offerings are scarcer than cold remedies with just one ingredient. Instead, the cold-war arsenal on pharmacy shelves is loaded with shotgun remedies.

Shotgun cold remedies usually contain two basic drugs, an antihistamine and a decongestant. Brands with just these two include *Contac, Drixoral* syrup, *Dimetapp,* and *Triaminic.* Other popular brands add pain reliever as a third ingredient—*Alka-Seltzer Plus, Benadryl Plus, Dimetapp Plus,* and *Dristan.*

The more drugs, the more symptoms a shotgun product can claim to treat. *Dristan,* a three-barrel remedy, claims success against 12 different cold symptoms: sinus pain, body aches, chills, fever, headache, sneezing, runny nose, watery eyes, postnasal drip, sinus congestion, nasal congestion, and sore throat.

Proponents say such remedies are economical and convenient: Just one purchase relieves all your symptoms. Most cold experts, however, consider the products to be irrational.

People differ greatly in their cold symptoms. Some suffer the whole gamut, while others escape with a mild runny nose and sneezes. As a result, users of shotgun remedies often pay for unnecessary drugs that increase the risk of side effects. Even when the drugs match the symptoms, the fixed doses in shotgun remedies may be inappropriate—inadequate for severe symptoms, too potent for mild ones.

The FDA's cold-remedy panel urged that cold remedies be limited to no more than three different drugs. It was "highly unlikely," the panel found, that anyone would need any more than that.

But the FDA overruled its panel, allowing manufacturers to load as many drugs as possible into their concoctions. Vick's *NyQuil,* America's leading cold remedy, contains five different drugs: an antihistamine, a

SELECTED COLD REMEDIES

With the exception of codeine, all brands listed below contain a single active ingredient helpful against a specific cold symptom. Most of the ingredients are also available as generic products or store brands.

Symptom	Remedy	Ingredient	Products
Congestion	Topical decongestant	phenylephrine oxymetazoline xylometazoline	*Dristan, Neo-Synephrine, Sinex* *Afrin, Duration, Dristan Long-lasting Nasal Spray* *Neo-Synephrine II*
	Oral decongestant	pseudoephedrine	*Oramyl, Sudafed, Sudanyl*
Sore throat	Medicated lozenges and sprays	phenol compounds benzocaine hexylresorcinol menthol	*Chloraseptic Sore Throat Spray* *Spec-T Sore Throat Anesthetic Lozenges* *Sucrets* *N'Ice Sugarless Cough Lozenges*
Headache, muscle aches, and fever	Pain reliever	aspirin acetaminophen ibuprofen	*Bayer, Bufferin, Norwich, St. Joseph Aspirin* *Datril, Tylenol* *Advil, Nuprin*
Coughs	Cough suppressant	dextromethorphan codeine diphenhydramine menthol	*Benylin DM, Delsym, Dr. Drake's, Pertussin 8-Hour Cough Formula, PediaCare 1 Liquid, St. Joseph Cough Syrup for Children, Hold 4-Hour Cough Suppressant* *Cheracol, Histadyl EC, Naldecon CX, Novahistine DH* *Benylin* *N'Ice Sugarless Cough Lozenges*
	Expectorant	guaifenesin	*Cotrex, 2/G, Hytuss, Nortussin, Robitussin*

decongestant, a pain reliever, a cough suppressant, and a stiff dose of alcohol. (It's 50 proof, comparable to crème de menthe or triple sec.) Other five-barrel specials include *Comtrex, CoTylenol,* and *Robitussin Night Relief.*

Presumably, if you can withstand the soporific effect of the antihistamine or alcohol, something in the mélange might work. But a more rational approach is to look for effective single-ingredient drugs. That way you can target just the symptoms you have, when you have them, and adjust the dose to fit their severity. The following table gives examples of the types of single-ingredient products to use for specific symptoms.

Decongestants Most cold sufferers experience nasal congestion, caused by swelling of the mucous membranes in the nose. Decongestants can ease that problem. They constrict dilated blood vessels, shrinking the swollen tissue and opening nasal passages. The result is freer breathing, better drainage, and reduced stuffiness.

There are two kinds of decongestants: topical (sprays and drops) and oral (tablets and caplets). Each has advantages and drawbacks.

Topical decongestants are more effective than oral ones. A recent study, for example, showed that the topical ingredient oxymetazoline produced four times as much decongestion as oral use of pseudoephedrine, the ingredient in *Sudafed* and several other oral products. The topical remedy also worked faster, producing improvement within five minutes versus 30 to 60 minutes for the oral decongestant.

Most standard topical decongestants—*Dristan, Sinex, Neo-Synephrine*—use phenylephrine hydrochloride as their active ingredient. Newer, long-acting products, such as *Afrin, Duration,* and *Neo-Synephrine II,* contain oxymetazoline or xylometazoline.

The drawback of topical decongestants is that overuse can lead to "rebound congestion," stuffiness worse than the original problem. Each application produces an initial decongestant effect and then some irritation and inflammation, which tends to go unnoticed. But if the drug is used frequently, the delayed effects begin to predominate. The more you use the product, the more irritated, inflamed, and blocked up your nasal passages become. Eventually, treatment may require the use of oral or topical steroid drugs to break the cycle. Accordingly, topical decongestants should be used sparingly, and only for a few days.

Probably the best time to use a topical decongestant is before bed, to help ensure a good night's sleep. Another good time is first thing in the morning, when nasal passages tend to be stuffiest.

In contrast to topical decongestants, oral ones can be taken daily for up to a week. They can be used alone or along with a topical product, serving as maintenance therapy to reduce the need for the topical decongestant.

Oral decongestants don't produce rebound congestion, but they can cause other side effects, such as mouth dryness or interference with sleep (if taken shortly before bedtime). A potentially more serious problem that can occur with their use is blood-pressure elevation.

The oral decongestant most likely to raise blood pressure is phenylpropanolamine (PPA). It's widely used in shotgun cold remedies (*Alka-Seltzer Plus, Contac, Dimetapp,* and *Dristan Capsules,* among others). In addition, it's the active ingredient in all diet pills, such as *Appedrine, Dexatrim,* and *Dietac.*

In 1984, an article in the *Journal of the American Medical Association* warned that PPA can produce severe or even life-threatening hypertension—at a dose only three times higher than its maximum recommended dose. Such a narrow difference between recommended and toxic doses was called "unique among over-the-counter drugs."

In January 1986, the FDA announced it would decide "in the near future" whether PPA was safe for OTC use. At this writing, the agency has yet to announce its verdict. In the meantime, anyone with high blood pressure should avoid products with PPA. People taking both diet pills and cold remedies may be exposing themselves to double jeopardy.

Pseudoephedrine, another popular oral decongestant, is a safer alternative. You can find it in many shotgun remedies or in single-ingredient decongestants such as *Sudafed, Sudanyl,* and *Oramyl.* Cheaper generic versions are also available.

Decongestants won't help a runny nose—and may possibly exacerbate the discomfort by enhancing drainage. Atropine, a seldom-used prescription drug, might offer some help. But for the most part, the war on runny noses must be waged with facial tissue.

Pain Relievers   About 25 percent of people with colds get headaches, 10 percent have muscle pain, and 1 percent run mild fevers. All these symptoms respond well to the three standard nonprescription pain relievers: aspirin, acetaminophen, and ibuprofen.

Aspirin and acetaminophen can be found in many shotgun cold remedies. But it's cheaper to buy the straight pain reliever.

As previously mentioned (see Chapter 1), children with cold symptoms shouldn't take aspirin because of its possible link with Reye's syndrome. Give them acetaminophen instead.

Vitamin Therapy   In 1970, interest in the therapeutic qualities of vitamin C was sparked with the publication of Linus Pauling's book *Vitamin C and the Common Cold.* Pauling cited several experimental studies, anecdotal evidence, and personal experience to support his belief that large doses of vitamin C can prevent or cure the common cold and possibly other respiratory infections as well.

After careful scrutiny, *The Medical Letter* and CU's medical consultants and statisticians concluded that the studies cited were inadequately controlled. At least 16 well-controlled studies since then have likewise failed to substantiate any beneficial effect of vitamin C in preventing or curing colds. A series of studies conducted in Toronto in the mid-1970s suggested that regular intake of about 120 milligrams of vitamin C daily—roughly the amount of eight ounces of orange juice—might reduce the general malaise of a cold, but the benefit was relatively minor. Megadoses of vitamin C can be harmful to some people—pregnant women and their fetuses, older people, and those with certain illnesses, for example—and, at high enough levels, even to the medically "normal" person.

According to the FDA advisory panel on cough and cold products, labels claiming that vitamins—alone or in combination with other products—are effective as cold preventives or cures should not be permitted. Furthermore, the panel recommended that vitamin C be dropped from OTC cold preparations unless and until appropriate studies have proved its effectiveness. (See Chapter 15 for more on vitamins.)

COUGH REMEDIES

Coughs afflict nearly half the people with colds and are sometimes the most troublesome of all cold symptoms. Syrups, tablets, and lozenges provide varying degrees of relief. Coughs that are most likely to warrant treatment are the dry, hacking kind that interfere with sleep.

But suppressing a cough isn't always a good idea. People with certain lung problems, such as chronic bronchitis, or emphysema, should be cautious about using cough suppressants. Coughing is the body's way of clearing secretions, irritants, and foreign matter from the lungs and throat. This protective reflex is triggered by a cough-control center in the brain, which responds to irritation. People with lung diseases often must expel excessive secretions and therefore should use cough suppressants only under medical supervision.

The FDA has approved three cough suppressants—drugs that directly inhibit the brain's cough reflex—as safe and effective: codeine, dextromethorphan, and diphenhydramine.

Codeine   Codeine is to coughs as aspirin is to headaches, the standard against which any alternative drug is compared. Although codeine is a narcotic, it rarely causes physical dependence when taken for a short time. In some states, it can be sold without a prescription.

Under Federal law, OTC codeine products must also include one or more nonnarcotic active ingredients. As a result, such cough preparations are all shotgun products. Examples include *Cheracol, Histadyl EC, Naldecon CX,* and *Novahistine DH.*

Dextromethorphan   Another cough suppressant, dextromethorphan, is widely available in syrups, tablets, and lozenges. Like codeine, it acts on the central nervous system to depress the cough reflex. Dextromethorphan is similar to codeine in effectiveness and is not addictive. Its efficacy and safety make it the best choice for suppressing a cough.

Although most products containing dextromethorphan are shotgun remedies, there are some cough syrups and lozenges with dextromethorphan as their sole active ingredient. The syrups include *Benylin DM, Delsym, Dr. Drake's, Pertussin 8-Hour Cough Formula, PediaCare 1 Liquid,* and *St. Joseph Cough Syrup for Children.* Lozenges offering just dextromethorphan are *Sucrets Cough Control Formula* and *Hold 4-Hour Cough Suppressant.*

Diphenhydramine   The third cough suppressant, diphenhydramine, appears to be used only in *Benylin Cough Syrup*. Diphenhydramine is an antihistamine that often causes drowsiness (it's the active ingredient in such sleep-aid products as *Sominex 2* and *Nytol*). So *Benylin* is best reserved for bedtime use.

Menthol and Camphor Two ingredients, menthol and camphor, quiet coughs by acting locally on the throat, not on the brain's cough center. The FDA concluded that their vapors have an anesthetic or analgesic effect. The most familiar product of this type is *Vicks Vapo-Rub*. Lozenges with more than five milligrams of menthol may similarly ease coughs.

Expectorants Another class of ingredients used for coughs is expectorants. They supposedly help liquefy and loosen phlegm, making it easier to cough up.

Expectorants have been widely used for years without much evidence that they work. But the FDA is expected to announce that new clinical data show that one expectorant—guaifenesin—is effective.

Guaifenesin is the staple ingredient in *Robitussin,* the nation's leading line of cough remedies. Plain *Robitussin* contains just guaifenesin. But several *Robitussin* products, as well as other brands, combine guaifenesin with a cough suppressant.

CU's medical consultants believe it makes poor sense to mix an expectorant—intended to make phlegm easier to cough up—with a drug that suppresses coughing. People who feel they might benefit from an expectorant would do better to choose a product with that alone. Such brands include *Colrex Expectorant, 2/G, Hytuss* tablets, and *Nortussin,* as well as plain *Robitussin.*

Ample fluid intake can also help loosen phlegm. Cough sufferers should try to consume about three or four pints of fluid a day, including the traditional sovereign remedy, chicken soup. Humidifying the air with a vaporizer may also help.

SORE THROAT REMEDIES

A sore throat is often the first symptom of a cold. It affects about half of all cold sufferers, who can choose from a legion of lozenges, sprays, and mouthwashes to soothe the pain.

The FDA considers seven ingredients effective in relieving or dulling sore-throat irritation: benzocaine, benzyl alcohol, dyclonine hydrochloride, hexylresorcinol, menthol, phenol compounds, and salicyl alcohol. Brands with sufficient amounts of these ingredients include *Chloraseptic Sore Throat* lozenges and spray, *Oracin, Spec-T Sore Throat Anesthetic Lozenges,* and *Sucrets.*

How well do mouthwashes and gargles relieve the pain of sore throat? Some gargles may provide temporary relief from inflammatory pain, although we know of no adequately controlled studies that have tested these observations. In fact, the simple act of gargling may bring some relief to the inflamed throat, independent of the specific composition of the gargling solution.

Warm salt water (one-half teaspoon of table salt to an eight-ounce glass of warm water) is useful as both a gargle and a mouthwash. In addition to the potentially beneficial effect of gargling, this mildly concentrated salt solution may help to reduce painful swelling.

What about aspirin gargles? The FDA found insufficient evidence that aspirin, when used topically, can relieve pain. In addition, aspirin can irritate inflamed mucous membranes.

Since dry indoor air can aggravate a sore throat, consider using a humidifier. There are now three basic types of humidifiers: electrolytic (steam) vaporizers, cool-mist, and ultrasonic. Whether the moisture is warm or cool makes no therapeutic difference. However, a steam vaporizer poses a risk of accidental shock or burn. A cool-mist model, on the other hand, requires more maintenance; the reservoir must be cleaned thoroughly before each use to eliminate the possibility of spraying droplets contaminated with bacteria or fungi into the air. The newer ultrasonic models pose no threat of burns and minimal threat of shocks, they greatly reduce the possibility of spreading molds and bacteria from the water reservoir (but should still be cleaned regularly), and they're virtually silent. Naturally, they are also the most expensive.

If your sore throat lasts more than a day or two, or is accompanied by a fever, check with a physician to find out if an exam is needed.

Keep in mind that all these remedies, no matter how effective, only relieve cold symptoms. The infection runs its course unimpeded by any of them. If your symptoms are severe, take it easy and stay home for a day or so. That might help protect others from catching your cold.

3

Allergy Treatment— and Mistreatment

Unsuspecting allergy victims have more to fear than just an allergen. They may also be victimized by those who would rush to treat their condition. Abuses include the overuse of allergy tests and shots, mail-order diagnosis, and the treatment of nonexistent food allergies. If you have allergies, as an estimated one out of five Americans do, learn the truth about the problem and what really helps before you fall for a questionable cure.

THE CAUSE OF ALLERGIES: IMMUNITY GONE HAYWIRE

The tendency to become sensitized to allergens is largely inherited. Symptoms can range from merely annoying to life-threatening. Most sufferers have hay fever, or "allergic rhinitis." Less-common problems include asthma, skin diseases such as atopic eczema, and food allergies. Symptoms vary, but the underlying cause is the same—a glitch in the body's immune defenses. The immune system protects against disease-causing germs, such as bacteria and viruses. But allergic people have an immune system that also reacts to harmless material, such as pollen, as if it were a threat.

Initial encounters with an allergen may prompt your immune system to form antibodies, which deploy on specialized cells called mast cells. When coated with antibodies, mast cells are like mines bristling with detonators. Millions of them lie in the respiratory and digestive tracts and in the skin, waiting for the right allergen to come along. When one does, the mast cells explode, releasing powerful chemicals such as histamine. These chemicals engage the "invader" but can also inflame nearby tissues, cause hives to form and airways to narrow, and stimulate mucus production in the nose and sinuses.

Usually, this reaction causes symptoms of hay fever, such as watery or itchy eyes, sneezing fits, and a runny or stuffy nose. (Despite the name, sufferers do not react to hay and do not run a fever.) The main culprits are pollens: primarily from trees in spring, grasses in early summer, and ragweed in late summer and early fall.

SELF-TREATMENT WITH OTC REMEDIES

Many allergic people have seasonal hay fever. Those who suffer from mild symptoms can try to ward off the allergy-producing substance (or substances) by installing an air conditioner or taking a well-timed vacation to a pollen-free area. If the first option isn't effective and the second one isn't feasible, some comfort may be found in a carefully selected over-the-counter (OTC) remedy or two, most likely an antihistamine and possibly a decongestant.

Antihistamines   Antihistamines are the mainstay of hay fever treatment, indeed providing rapid temporary relief to most sufferers. They act by preventing histamine from exerting its noxious effects. Some antihistamines also have a drying effect on nasal secretions.

While OTC antihistamines rarely cause serious side effects in teenagers and adults, drowsiness is a common complaint. That makes their use undesirable when you need to be alert, and dangerous when you drive a car or operate machinery. Using antihistamines in combination with alcohol, tranquilizers, or other central nervous system depressants magnifies their sedative effect and can be hazardous.

Some people develop a tolerance to this side effect after using antihistamines for a while. If drowsiness is a problem, try taking the antihistamine only at bedtime at first and then increase the dosage by cautiously introducing daytime medication over the course of the first week.

Certain types of antihistamines are more likely than others to produce drowsiness in the first place. The table on page 33 lists dosages for safe and effective antihistamines, as recommended by the U.S. Food and Drug Administration (FDA) advisory panel on OTC cough, cold, and allergy products. Of the three main chemical classes of antihistamines listed in the table, the *alkylamines* generally have the least sedative effect and the *ethanolamines* the most. The *ethylenediamines* fall somewhere between. (Phenindamine tartrate, a compound with a different chemical structure from the others, commonly stimulates rather than sedates.)

While those chemical groupings may be useful as a general guide, the side effects of antihistamines can vary widely from one individual to the next. You might be knocked out by an alkylamine and function very well on an ethylenediamine; someone else might react just the opposite. You may need to experiment with different products in different chemical classes to find the most suitable one.

CU's medical consultants suggest confining experimentation to those OTC products containing one of the antihistamines listed in our table at its recommended dosage level. At this time, *Chlor-Trimeton, Dimetane, Novahistine,* and *Pfeiffer Allergy Tablets* are among the brand-name products that meet those ingredient and dosage requirements. Before making a purchase, ask a pharmacist whether any of the antihistamines listed in our table is available as a generic product that can save you money.

Once a satisfactory antihistamine has been found, you may discover that the product no longer works after a while. Just as it is possible to develop a tolerance to the drug's sedative quality, it is also possible to become tolerant to its therapeutic effect. If that happens, switch to another antihistamine.

Curiously, children sometimes react to antihistamine use with insomnia and stimulation of the central nervous system rather than with drowsiness. Because of antihistamines' less-predictable effects on children, anyone aged 6 to 12 should be given these drugs with caution. They should not be given to children under six except with the advice and supervision of a physician. Pregnant and lactating women, men with urinary problems, and people with asthma, glaucoma, or convulsive disorders should consult a physician before using antihistamines.

Decongestants An antihistamine is most effective if used before allergy symptoms become severe. But even then, it usually doesn't work well against a stuffy nose. So a hay fever sufferer may also need a decongestant, which can be taken either orally in pill or liquid form, or topically as nasal sprays or drops. The topical decongestants should be used cautiously—if at all—for hay fever, because treatment may be needed for

RECOMMENDED DOSAGES OF SAFE AND EFFECTIVE ANTIHISTAMINES

Antihistamine	Dosage			
	Adults	Children 6 to 12 Years	Children 2* to 6 Years
The following three antihistamines are alkylamines, which tend to cause less drowsiness than most others:			
Brompheniramine maleate	4 mg every 4–6 hrs	2 mg every 4–6 hrs	1 mg every 4–6 hrs
Chlorpheniramine maleate	4 mg every 4–6 hrs	2 mg every 4–6 hrs	1 mg every 4–6 hrs
Pheniramine maleate	12.5–25 mg every 4–6 hrs	6.25–12 mg every 4–6 hrs	3.125–6.25 mg every 4–6 hrs
The following two antihistamines are ethylenediamines, which tend to cause somewhat more drowsiness than those listed above:			
Pyrilamine maleate	25–50 mg every 6–8 hrs	12.2–25 mg every 6–8 hrs	6.25–12.5 mg every 6–8 hrs
Thonzylamine hydrochloride	50–100 mg every 4–6 hrs	25–50 mg every 4–6 hrs	12.5–25 mg every 4–6 hrs
The following antihistamine is an ethanolamine, and tends to cause somewhat more drowsiness than those listed above:			
Doxylamine succinate	7.5–12.5 mg every 4–6 hrs	3.75–6.25 mg every 4–6 hrs	(Consult physician)
The following antihistamine tends to have a stimulant effect rather than a sedative one:			
Phenindamine tartrate	25 mg every 4–6 hrs	12.5 mg every 4–6 hrs	6.25 mg every 4–6 hrs

*There is no recommended dosage for children under two, except with the advice and supervision of a physician.

many weeks and frequent use leads to dependency and "rebound conges-tion." People with high blood pressure, heart disease, diabetes, thyroid disease, or urinary problems should consult a physician before using any decongestant. (Safe and effective decongestants are discussed in more detail in Chapter 2, pages 24–25.)

Because hay fever sufferers often use both decongestants and antihis-tamines, the two drugs are sold in combination in many OTC allergy products. Among combination products, *Chlor-Trimeton Decongestant, Dimetapp, Fedahist, Ryna, Sudafed Plus,* and *Triaminic* currently offer effective dosages of one recommended decongestant and one recom-mended antihistamine. Again, less-expensive generic versions may be available.

While taking a fixed-combination product may be more convenient than separate medications, it locks you into dosages that may not be exactly right. For example, if you are adequately medicated with less anti-histamine, you might want to reduce the dose to alleviate drowsiness. But cutting down on the antihistamine dose would mean also reducing the decongestant dose—and perhaps rendering it totally ineffective. And since a stuffy nose might not *always* accompany the other symptoms, you would be medicating a nonexistent symptom if you took a combination product whenever hay fever flared up. Because of such drawbacks, CU's medical consultants suggest using each medication separately—at least until you have confirmed the individual ingredients and dosages that are right for you.

Shotgun Remedies Most OTC cold and allergy products include far more than two ingredients. These "shotgun remedies" may boast five or more, possibly including caffeine, one or more painkillers, an anticholin-ergic (a drying agent) such as atropine sulfate or belladonna alkaloids, among others. Of these additions, only a painkiller might make sense—but even then, not every time. Some hay fever victims do sometimes suf-fer headaches, but this is rarely an ongoing symptom. As with antihista-mine and decongestant, you'd be much better off taking the pain-reliever component separately, and only as needed (see Chapter 1).

CU's medical consultants believe the heavily advertised "timed-release" or "sustained-action" cold and hay fever products (including

Contac and *Dristan* capsules) should be avoided not only because of what's in them, but because of the unpredictable rate at which they work in any given individual. If the ingredients are released too slowly, there may be no therapeutic effect. If they are released too quickly, side effects may increase in number and severity.

Even if a satisfactory OTC product for your allergy is found, be on the alert for complications. Pain or popping sounds in the ear may indicate a problem that could cause vertigo (an unbalanced spinning sensation often accompanied by nausea) and eventually lead to hearing loss. Pain above the teeth, in the cheeks, above the eyes, or on the side of the nose could indicate a bacterial sinus infection. Persistent coughing, difficulty in breathing, and wheezing may signal asthma, a more serious allergic ailment than hay fever. If any of these symptoms occurs, see a physician.

SEEKING PROFESSIONAL TREATMENT

Some people need more than an OTC remedy. They may suffer debilitating hay fever symptoms for months on end or even year-round. Or they may have asthma aggravated by allergies, or even life-threatening reactions to certain insect stings. They require professional help.

Whatever the problem, the critical first step is a thorough medical history. The series of questions—what are your symptoms, when and where do they occur, and so on—may reveal that your problems actually arise from something other than an allergy. Often symptoms may stem from a respiratory infection, tobacco smoke, or some other nonallergic cause. If you do have allergies, the history can narrow the possibilities. Seasonal symptoms, for example, suggest that one or more pollens are at fault. Recurring symptoms may point to some factor at home or work, such as mold, dust, or pets.

A diagnostic test may also be needed to pin down the allergy. Most commonly used is a skin test, which detects antibodies your body has developed against specific allergens. Typically, using the "scratch test" method, the doctor or assistant uses a penlike instrument to make a series of pricks on your back or forearm. A drop of allergen extract is then placed on each puncture. Many different allergens can be tested in this manner. Alternatively, some specialists prefer to inject the extract directly into the skin (intradermal skin test). A positive test produces a small, circular welt around the puncture or injection site within 10 to 20 minutes. The bigger the welt, the greater the sensitivity to the allergen.

Once an allergy has been identified, the most effective way to treat it is to avoid what causes it. With pollen, of course, that's usually not possible—although an air conditioner may help keep it out of the house. For many other allergens, an allergist will recommend avoidance *before* trying any other treatment. If your cat makes you wheeze, no treatment can rival giving it away. If you react to house dust, removing bedroom rugs and putting mattresses and pillows in zippered, airtight covers may ease the problem. A dehumidifier can help rid your basement of mold.

When avoidance isn't possible, the next-best solution is to relieve symptoms. If OTC antihistamines and decongestants aren't helpful, an allergist may prescribe other drugs. During the last 10 years, new prescription drugs with reduced side effects have enhanced allergy treatment significantly. Here's a brief rundown of the most important ones:

Terfenadine (Seldane) Introduced in 1985, this is the first of a new breed of antihistamines that seldom cause drowsiness. Its disadvantage is that it costs much more than OTC antihistamines at present. Competition may lower its price tag. By 1990, the FDA is expected to approve two other nonsedating antihistamines: astemizole (Hismanal) and loratadine (Claritin). Both are longer-acting than terfenadine—which may soon become available over-the-counter.

Cromolyn Sodium (Nasalcrom) This liquid nasal spray is quite effective in preventing symptoms of both asthma and hay fever. (It should *not* be used to treat an acute asthma attack; it could make matters worse.) Cromolyn appears to toughen mast cells, making them less likely to break apart and release histamine when confronted with an appropriate allergen. It is notable for its lack of side effects.

Steroid Nasal Sprays Containing either beclomethasone dipropionate (Vancenase, Beconase) or flunisolide (Nasalide), these are especially effective against nasal congestion. While their action is not immediate, it is limited to their target area—the nose and bronchial passages—which minimizes the risk of side effects that can occur with other dosage forms of steroids.

Optimal treatment may require a combination of drugs—for instance, an antihistamine to help watery, itchy eyes and a steroid spray for nasal congestion. Such therapy can usually relieve symptoms in all but the most severe cases.

THE SHOT DOCTORS

Although they have their place in allergy therapy, injections are perhaps the most overused and misused treatment. In recent years, their popularity has been boosted by the proliferation of mail-order allergy laboratories around the country. These labs will analyze a blood sample to identify the patient's supposed allergies and send a printout of the results back to the doctor, who can then order extracts to use in allergy shots.

A blood test is more expensive and less sensitive than a skin test, which should be performed only by a trained allergist. The main advantage of a blood test is that it requires just a single puncture, making it more acceptable for toddlers and for people with extensive skin disease.

However, mail-order diagnosis is tempting to some doctors with little or no training in allergy. It offers a simple way to treat allergic patients by administering shots instead of recommending drugs or referring them to specialists. (After all, patients treated with shots return to the doctor's office much more frequently than those on prescription drugs.)

But mail-order diagnoses may be inaccurate or misleading. An erroneous diagnosis can lead to costly and potentially hazardous treatment—a series of shots that will set you back several hundred dollars a year for two or more years. And even with an accurate diagnosis, allergy shots are rarely appropriate treatment. They're unnecessary for most hay fever victims, and they don't work at all against food allergies.

Too many patients are put on shots simply because they have positive skin or blood tests. Often these people don't even have a history of allergy to the putative antigen. What's more, overzealous skin-testing can increase the chances of a false positive result. Indeed, some doctors give an excessive number of skin tests, sometimes performing 100 or more in a single visit—a practice that coincidentally escalates their fees. The American Medical Association's Council on Scientific Affairs recently stated that the number of skin tests "should rarely exceed 50."

Even significant allergies may not warrant shots. For example, a skin test may suggest you're extremely sensitive to Bermuda grass. But that's a problem only if you live in or visit an area where Bermuda grass is prevalent. If you don't, you surely don't need shots.

The Time for Shots

When an allergy has been accurately diagnosed, treatment with drugs has fallen short, and avoidance of the allergen is impractical, the patient may indeed be a candidate for allergy shots. The shots can be effective against some allergens you inhale—such as pollens that cause hay fever or aggravate asthma—and against allergies to insect stings.

Treatment begins with shots once or twice a week. The first injection contains a very dilute antigen dose, so as not to provoke an allergic reaction, such as generalized itching or hives. Each succeeding shot contains a higher concentration of the allergen. The aim is to increase the concentration gradually to a maintenance dose—the highest concentration that the patient can tolerate without an allergic reaction. That process commonly takes from four to six months. After that, the patient receives monthly injections of the maintenance dose, generally for at least two years.

One of the major abuses involving allergy shots—even when shots are likely to be appropriate—is treatment that lasts too long. You should expect to see improvement after one year, or two years at most. Shots that don't produce an improvement within two years should be discontinued. When shots do work, they should be kept up for three to five years, after which they usually can be stopped. For about half the patients, relief from symptoms will persist indefinitely. If symptoms recur, another course of shots can always be undertaken.

Allergy shots can work well when used appropriately. But even in the right situation, shots have drawbacks that should make them the treatment of last resort. First of all, they contain allergens, so there's always the risk of an allergic reaction. A patient receiving shots walks a fine line: Improvements are greatest at the highest maintenance dose, but that's also the dose most likely to cause allergic reactions. In very rare cases, such reactions can be fatal.

Second, allergy shots pose a danger because of the uncertain quality of their extracts. In contrast to other types of drugs, most allergenic extracts lack uniform standards of potency, and in some instances the differences can be significant. The dust extract sold by one company, for instance, may be as much as 1000 times stronger than a similar extract sold by another. That could be dangerous, especially if the doctor were to switch from a weaker to a stronger extract in the course of treatment.

So far, only about a dozen of the 1500 different extracts on the market have been standardized. They include some of the most important ones, however, such as short ragweed, several grasses, cat, and house-dust mites (the major allergen in house dust).

Which Extracts Work?

In 1974, the FDA convened a panel of allergy experts to review the efficacy of extracts. In 1985, the panel concluded that many of the 1500 marketed extracts were effective for diagnostic use in skin tests. Their value in *treatment,* however, was far less certain. The panel found convincing proof of efficacy for only a handful of extracts, including ragweed, certain grasses, mountain cedar, and dust mites. They reasoned that extracts of other inhaled allergens would probably work also.

Here's the current status of some commonly used extracts:

Ragweed   Most immunotherapy research has looked at ragweed, the major cause of hay fever. Well-controlled studies show that shots for ragweed pollen work for about 85 percent of patients.

Pollens   While clinical studies are lacking for many pollens, such as birch, oak, red maple, annual bluegrass, and others, most authorities believe that pollen extracts are effective.

House Dust   While some allergists say these extracts work, others strongly disagree. The raw materials for several such extracts come from the contents of vacuum-cleaner bags, with no consistency from one batch to another. Analyses show that the extracts contain anything from dog and cat dander to allergens associated with dust mites, rodent hairs, molds, and other substances. The FDA advisory panel concluded that house-dust extracts are potentially unsafe and should be taken off the market, but the FDA has not yet acted on the panel's recommendation.

Mold A few studies that evaluated mold extracts produced inconclusive results. CU's allergy consultants said they prefer to treat mold allergies with drugs whenever possible.

Cats An estimated 58 million cats live in 27 million American homes, and many people are allergic to them. Until recently, researchers thought the problem was mainly cat dander. Now they know that most people allergic to cats are also sensitive to the saliva cats apply to themselves when grooming. Three clinical studies have shown that while shots allow people to tolerate cats for longer periods before symptoms hit, many of these people remain quite sensitive. While cat-extract shots may help people who are exposed to cats occasionally, perhaps when visiting cat owners, such shots are totally ineffective for allergic people who live with cats. For those people, the most effective measure is to find another home for the cat—or at least keep it out of the bedroom.

Insects For people who experience serious reactions from insect stings, studies show that allergy shots afford almost complete protection against harmful effects from subsequent stings.

ASTHMA AND ALLERGIES

Should asthmatics get allergy shots? Some doctors think so, but such treatment remains controversial. Many of America's 15 million asthmatics do have allergies—about half the adults and 90 percent of children. Many people with adult-onset asthma, which can be quite debilitating, have no allergies at all. When allergies do provoke asthma, avoidance is still the best treatment. Pets and dust often cause problems; removing them may provide relief.

Today's drugs, the second line of defense, usually control the wheezing, coughing, and shortness of breath that occur with asthma. Bronchodilators, for example, make breathing easier by widening bronchial tubes that have been narrowed by muscle spasm, inflammation, and mucus. Asthmatics with minimal wheezing may often obtain short-term relief with OTC bronchodilator inhalers containing epinephrine and similar drugs. Longer-acting bronchodilator sprays that require a prescription include those containing albuterol or terbutaline. Theophylline, another long-acting bronchodilator, can be taken orally. Oral forms of albuterol and terbutaline are also available. Other prescription drugs that alleviate asthma include the steroid and cromolyn sprays described on page 36. (To avoid masking a worsening asthmatic condition, bronchodilators should be used only under the supervision of a physician.)

Some asthmatics—those not helped by avoidance or drugs and whose attacks are serious enough to require hospitalization—might be candidates for allergy shots. But their allergies must first be documented. Asthma can be triggered by many factors besides allergies, including exercise, stress, respiratory infections, cold weather, and cigarette smoke. Current evidence suggests that shots may be worth a try in carefully chosen asthma patients, particularly those with allergies to grasses and cats.

FOOD ALLERGIES AND INTOLERANCES

Pop-medicine publications have spread the word that food allergies are a major public-health problem, causing myriad physical and psychological symptoms. Actually, true food allergies, in which a food provokes an immune response, are uncommon. Only about 5 percent of children and less than 2 percent of adults have well-documented food allergies.

What people call food allergies are often food intolerances. Some of those are individual idiosyncrasies without a detectable physical basis. Millions of Americans report such idiosyncrasies and get along simply by avoiding the offending food. But some food intolerances arise from well-identified causes. Many people have trouble with milk, for example, because they're deficient in an enzyme needed to digest lactose (milk sugar). They may experience bloating, diarrhea, or other gastrointestinal symptoms from milk, ice cream, and other dairy products.

The distinction between food intolerance and food allergy is important. People with a true food allergy must avoid the offending food in any quantity and at all times. But those with a mild food intolerance may be able to eat small to moderate amounts of a problem food with little discomfort. Mistaking a food intolerance for a food allergy can needlessly restrict what you eat and even result in nutritional deficiencies.

The main culprits in true food allergies are cow's milk protein, egg whites, various kinds of nuts, and, especially, seafood. If you're allergic to any of them, you might experience one or more of several symptoms: nausea, vomiting, diarrhea, rashes, itching, difficulty breathing. In rare cases, even fatal reactions can occur. (Patients with proven food allergies are commonly advised to carry a preloaded epinephrine syringe to take in case of a severe reaction.) There's no scientific evidence, however, that food allergies cause psychological or behavioral problems.

If you think you have a food allergy, you should be referred to a physician who is board-certified as an allergist (one who has passed the examination administered by the American Board of Allergy and Immunology). You may receive skin tests using food extracts. A positive test result requires confirmation, through either a well-documented history of allergic reactions to the food or a controlled oral "challenge," in which the suspect food is served under the supervision of a physician. If you do have a food allergy, the allergist will tell you there is only one effective treatment: Avoid the food. Shots, a qualified allergist will tell you, are totally useless as a therapy for food allergies.

But there are other physicians who contend that food allergies *can* be treated, often with extracts that you administer to yourself. Among those physicians are some otolaryngologists—ear, nose, and throat specialists. In recent years, about 20 percent of such specialists have turned to allergy treatment, calling themselves "otolaryngic allergists." Such self-styled allergists contend there's no limit to the insidious things a food can do to you. "The list of possible disorders that can be caused by food allergies is almost endless," declares a pamphlet published by the American Academy of Otolaryngic Allergy. "Even more startling," continues the pamphlet, "is the mounting evidence that foods and chemicals may cause severe difficulties in the nervous system and in the mind itself." But fortunately, it reassures, "most cases of food allergy can be helped" through the use of "modern procedures."

A second group of unorthodox allergy practitioners includes physicians of various types who call themselves clinical ecologists. They contend that not only foods but the chemicals around us trigger numerous physical and psychological problems. Otolaryngic allergists and clinical ecologists often use similar techniques for diagnosing and treating food allergies. One is the "intracutaneous provocative food test," in which the food extract is injected into the arm supposedly to provoke—and thereby detect—food allergy. Once a reaction has been provoked, a weaker solution of the extract is then injected to "neutralize" it. That neutralizing dose is then used for food-allergy treatment whenever the patient expects to confront the food and simply must eat some. A variation on this testing-and-treatment theme is the "sublingual" method, in which food extract drops are placed under the tongue instead of injected.

Several controlled studies have now evaluated those techniques for efficacy. All concluded that the measures are ineffective both for diagnosing and for treating food allergies. In 1983, the Health Care Financing Administration (HCFA) proposed to exclude both intracutaneous and sublingual methods from coverage under Medicare. The HCFA said both of the methods lacked "scientific evidence of effectiveness." The HCFA proposal prompted the otolaryngic allergists to begin a clinical study of those methods, which they'd been using uncritically since 1961. CU was allowed to look at the study before it was published. We asked two board-certified allergists familiar with allergy research to review it. They independently identified serious flaws in the study's research methods.

The California Medical Association, the American Academy of Allergy and Immunology, and a committee of the Ontario Ministry of Health have also assessed provocation testing and neutralization therapy. They all judged the techniques to be unproven. The American Academy of Allergy and Immunology described the techniques as having "no plausible rationale or immunologic basis."

In 1983, an FDA advisory panel on allergenic extracts concluded that food extracts are unsafe and ineffective for treating food allergy. Physicians can still use the extracts any way they want, because the FDA can't dictate medical practice. But unapproved use of a drug increases a physician's vulnerability in the event of a malpractice suit and may not be covered by insurance plans.

RECOMMENDATIONS

If you have reason to suspect hay fever and your symptoms are mild, you might experiment with OTC remedies, following the guidelines outlined earlier. An antihistamine and/or a decongestant may be all that you need to relieve seasonal symptoms. Then again, there may be no OTC remedy that gives *sufficient* relief. Or there may be side effects as distressing as the original symptoms. If you're not satisfied with the choice of nonprescription medications—or not sure you have hay fever—consult your physician. He or she may be able to help you identify and avoid your allergen, offer prescription drugs, or refer you to an allergist to evaluate your condition and possibly consider shot therapy.

But before resorting to shots for any allergy, a physician should first determine that:

- You've had the symptoms over a period of at least two years—long enough to indicate a chronic rather than a temporary problem.
- The symptoms disrupt your life. They're severe and persist for several weeks or months each year.
- Neither avoidance nor medication is effective.
- There is evidence that shots will work against your particular allergies.

Allergists do make exceptions and may choose to administer allergy shots without following such stringent guidelines. A singer, for instance, may need shots to be entirely free of symptoms. An airline pilot may want shots in order to avoid any sedating effects from drugs.

For most patients, though, drugs are preferable. They cost less; at an average of $20 per shot, a typical series of shots plus a consultation will come to about $400 a year. They are usually needed for only a few weeks or months each year. And they work faster; you can see results in a day or two versus a year or more for shots. Even when successful, shots may fail to provide complete relief; patients often need drug therapy as well.

If you're seeking help for allergies that can't be handled by OTC medications, check with your physician. He or she may recommend a visit to a board-certified allergist, who has received specialized training in treating such problems. You can ask your physician about the allergist's qualifications or you can call the American Board of Allergy and Immunology in Philadelphia (215-349-9466) for the information. In addition, the "Directory of Medical Specialists," which is available in the reference section of many public libraries, includes a listing of board-certified allergists.

Indigestion and Antacids

4

Americans spend close to one billion dollars a year on nonprescription digestive remedies—mostly for hundreds of antacids, including syrupy liquids, fizzing powders, and chewable tablets. All these products attempt to do the same thing: neutralize stomach acid.

What is "stomach acid" and why does it need to be neutralized? The cells that line the stomach secrete hydrochloric acid continuously, with greatest production shortly after meals. The acid helps dissolve food and activate pepsin, an enzyme that breaks down protein. But at certain times and under certain conditions, the acid causes a burning sensation.

The burning usually takes place not in the stomach but in the esophagus, the tube that carries food and liquid from the mouth to the stomach. A special muscle, or sphincter, between the esophagus and stomach usually keeps the stomach's caustic juices from "refluxing," or backing up, into the esophagus. But sometimes refluxing does occur, bringing stomach juice into contact with the sensitive lining of the lower esophagus.

The resulting discomfort has gone by different names through the years. Until the 1970s, antacid makers claimed their products relieved such miseries as "the blahs," "gassy-acid nausea," and morning sickness. Since then, however, the U.S. Food and Drug Administration (FDA) has forced manufacturers to tone down those claims. Now, antacid labels are all basically the same: "For the relief of heartburn, sour stomach, or acid indigestion, and upset stomach associated with these symptoms."

Actually, the terms *heartburn, sour stomach,* and *acid indigestion* all refer to the same basic symptom, with minor distinctions. Heartburn characteristically begins low in the front of the chest and may rise toward the throat. Acid indigestion and sour stomach are vaguer terms, but they often mean that stomach juice has entered the mouth, causing a burning sensation and taste. To simplify matters, most physicians use "heartburn" to describe all types of irritation caused by wayward stomach juice.

Many laypeople, however, lump these three terms, along with many other complaints, in the category of "upset stomach." As a result, antacid manufacturers may claim relief for upset stomach on their labels—as long as they specify that it's upset stomach *associated with* heartburn, acid indigestion, or sour stomach. That's to indicate that antacids probably won't help other types of stomach complaints, such as nausea, stomach-ache, abdominal cramps, and gas pains. Conversely, products that may help some of these other symptoms probably won't help heartburn.

UNDERSTANDING, PREVENTING, AND RELIEVING HEARTBURN

About 10 percent of the population has heartburn every day; another 30 percent experiences it occasionally. Women are affected more often than men.

Heartburn can range from barely noticeable, seemingly "normal" irritation to severe pain inside the chest. The intensity of the pain depends mainly on the amount of stomach juice reaching the esophagus, how caustic it is, and how long it stays there. In more severe cases, the acid damages the esophageal lining and causes inflammation (esophagitis), intense pain, difficulty in swallowing, even ulceration and bleeding.

Heartburn results most commonly from overeating and tends to occur about an hour after a large meal. It is often associated with specific foods, though any food may provoke heartburn in any individual at any time. Anxiety and stress, by triggering increased stomach acid production, can also bring on heartburn.

Antacids are the mainstay of heartburn treatment. They can be taken when symptoms begin or, as a preventive, 30 to 60 minutes after a meal you suspect may cause heartburn. An antacid generally reduces symptoms within three to five minutes after you take it. The effect lasts only about an hour, however, and the symptoms can then recur. To break this cycle, it is important to prevent the refluxing of stomach juice that causes heartburn.

Several steps can help. Certain foods are known to affect the sphincter that closes off the esophagus. Fatty foods, alcohol, and chocolate tend to relax the sphincter, opening the gate for the caustic juices to reflux from below. Conversely, a high-protein, low-fat diet helps to increase sphincter tone. So-called acid foods—tomato products and citrus juice—are also implicated in heartburn. They may irritate the esophagus directly, particularly in people who already have heartburn, thus making the condition worse.

Cigarettes are notorious for causing heartburn by lowering sphincter tone, most probably because of the nicotine. The role of coffee (both with and without caffeine) in heartburn is contradictory. It appears to increase sphincter tone, which is good, and also to increase acid production, which is bad. On balance, the bad probably outweighs the good, so the usual recommendation is to forgo coffee if you have a tendency to heartburn.

Gravity helps keep the stomach contents away from the esophagus, which explains why many heartburn sufferers are afflicted when they go to bed too soon after eating. One effective measure is to elevate the head of the bed at least six inches; a wedged pillow also works, but not as well. Avoiding meals or snacks before bedtime helps reduce the amount of acid secreted that can reflux and cause trouble. Heartburn sufferers should also try to avoid lying down or even bending over soon after a meal.

Increased abdominal pressure can also force stomach juices upward and bring on heartburn, as many pregnant women can attest. To lower abdominal pressure, lose weight if you're obese, do not engage in strenuous exercise, and avoid tight garments.

Related Problems: Ulcers and Gastritis

The bad effects of stomach acid are not limited to heartburn. Acid can damage the lining of the stomach or of the adjacent duodenum, the upper part of the small intestine. That can cause erosions (ulcers) or inflammation (gastritis or duodenitis). For many years, physicians have prescribed antacids for symptoms that arise from these problems. Studies have shown that antacids in high doses can help heal duodenal ulcers.

However, a new class of prescription drugs has emerged that can better treat many of these conditions. Known as histamine-2 blockers, or H2 blockers, these drugs—which include cimetidine (Tagamet), ranitidine (Zantac), famotidine (Pepcid), and nizatidine (Axid)—all interfere with the secretion of stomach acid from acid-producing cells. According to their FDA-approved indications (duodenal ulcer, benign gastric ulcer, pathological hypersecretory conditions), they are probably overused. But their popularity among physicians and patients attests to their relatively minor side effects—although the long-term effects of continuous blockade of stomach acid secretion remain to be seen.

Chronic antacid users may actually be trying to relieve one of these more serious problems rather than a persistent "upset stomach." That can be dangerous. While an antacid may relieve ulcer pain, the ulcer may occasionally get worse without your knowing it. Stomach cancers may also be mistaken for repeatedly upset stomach; the use of antacids to relieve pain may delay their detection. Anyone with stomach pain that recurs for more than two weeks should stop self-medication and consult a physician.

One problem often confused with indigestion has nothing whatever to do with the gastrointestinal tract. The pain of a heart attack can mimic simple indigestion. Features that distinguish a heart attack include a sensation of chest pressure or tightness rather than burning, sometimes radiating to the arms, neck, jaw, or upper back. Anyone experiencing such symptoms—often accompanied by sweating and weakness—should seek medical attention immediately.

JUDGING EFFECTIVENESS

Are antacids effective against heartburn? The many people who have found relief by downing two tablets or a tablespoonful no doubt think so. Specialists consulted by CU agreed—but said that their belief is based only on informal clinical observations, not on hard scientific evidence. To CU's knowledge, no well-controlled clinical trials with human subjects have been performed to determine whether antacids are more effective than placebos. One reason: The FDA review panel for antacid products never required that antacid manufacturers conduct such studies, but settled instead for a simple laboratory test.

The laboratory test required by the FDA resembles the familiar *Rolaids* commercial ("absorbs 47 times its weight in excess stomach acid"). Acid and antacid are mixed together in a glass beaker. For a product to qualify as an antacid, a standard dose must neutralize a certain amount of hydrochloric acid. For each brand, the total amount of acid neutralized is expressed as a number: the acid neutralizing capacity (ANC) per dose. Television ads often refer obliquely to the ANC: "Without its top layer, *Di-Gel* consumes as much heartburn-producing acid as plain antacids, like *Rolaids*"; "Compared to the leading tablet, *Tempo* is 75 percent stronger in acid-neutralizing power"; "*Lo-Sal* is twice as effective as the leading tablet."

But will *Di-Gel, Tempo,* and *Lo-Sal* really work better against heartburn than, say, *Rolaids,* which has a lower ANC? A test in a glass beaker can't determine the answer. The FDA recognizes the test's limitations and won't allow ANC values to appear on product labels. The agency fears that consumers might rely entirely on the numbers, when there's no clinical evidence that higher numbers mean greater effectiveness.

We tend to disagree with the FDA's judgment on antacid labeling and believe that ANC values should be available to consumers. They would provide one of the few ways to compare different antacid brands. But consumers would not rely on the numbers for efficacy, as this information would be useful only for comparing prices. Higher ANC values may not always be better in relieving symptoms than lower ones are; but of two brands that have the same ANC value, the one that costs less would be the better buy.

Tablets are more convenient to carry than a bottle, and more likely to be taken in the proper dosage. Suspensions, however, offer a compensating advantage. A teaspoon of the liquid generally has a higher acid neutralizing capacity than a tablet of the same brand.

The Ingredient Lineup

The hundreds of antacids on the shelves make choosing confusing. But there are basically just four active ingredients involved. Some products use one, others include two, and some even more. Unfortunately, the ingredients that are fastest-acting for occasional heartburn have drawbacks that often make them unsuitable for long-term use. These are the four:

Sodium Bicarbonate Ordinary baking soda. A potent neutralizer that reacts rapidly with stomach acid, it's probably the fastest-acting and cheapest antacid available. (Brands that currently contain sodium bicarbonate as their single active ingredient include *Alka-Seltzer Effervescent Antacid, Bell-Ans, Citrocarbonate,* and *Soda Mint.*)

Sodium bicarbonate is fine for occasional heartburn (defined as once a week or less). However, it is the least desirable antacid ingredient for frequent use, for one and possibly two reasons. It is highly alkaline and readily absorbed into the bloodstream; regular use may affect the body's acid-base balance and may encourage urinary tract infections by making the urine more alkaline. And the sodium component rules out its use by people on sodium-restricted diets.

Alka-Seltzer Effervescent Antacid contains citric acid, which buffers the sodium bicarbonate solution so that it's not as strongly alkaline (and which also helps to create the fizz). You can modify ordinary baking soda the same way—and make it taste better than *Alka-Seltzer*—by dissolving half a teaspoon of baking soda in half a glass of "natural" citic acid: orange juice. However, this doesn't reduce the high sodium content.

Calcium Carbonate This ingredient—the main component of chalk—shares some of the assets of sodium bicarbonate: It's inexpensive, reasonably fast-acting, and potent as an acid neutralizer. (Brands of calcium carbonate tablets include *Alka-Mints, Amitone, Calcium Rich Rolaids, Chooz, Dicarbosil, Titralac,* and *Tums.*)

These products are fine for occasional heartburn. In large doses over a prolonged period of time, however, they may raise calcium levels in the blood and urine, increasing the likelihood of kidney stones and impaired kidney function. This drawback prompted the FDA antacid panel to set a maximum recommended dose of eight grams of calcium carbonate daily (equal to 16 *Tums* tablets) for no more than two weeks. Unfortunately, many people exceed even that liberal recommendation. (For healthy people who have not experienced problems with kidney stones, an intake of one to 1½ grams of calcium daily from food and calcium supplements is a reasonable measure to help prevent osteoporosis, an abnormal loss of bone that can occur with age. See Chapter 21 for more on osteoporosis.)

Research has shown that calcium carbonate can cause "acid rebound" by triggering increased amounts of stomach acid after its own antacid effect has subsided. Whether acid rebound actually impairs calcium carbonate's overall clinical effectiveness as an antacid is not known. Constipation, which has traditionally been attributed to calcium carbonate, occurs only at high doses.

Magnesium Hydroxide Milk of magnesia, the common name for magnesium hydroxide, is a nearly perfect antacid. First, it's a good, fast-acting acid neutralizer. Second, frequent and long-term use is possible for most people. Those with kidney disease, however, are unable to eliminate magnesium adequately, allowing it to accumulate in the body and eventually cause serious problems.

Magnesium hydroxide's main drawback is its well-known laxative effect. The antacid dose is only one to three teaspoons, while the laxative dose is usually six teaspoons or more. But even the smaller dose can cause diarrhea in susceptible individuals or if doses are taken throughout the day.

Aluminum Hydroxide A few antacids have aluminum hydroxide—slow-acting and weak as an acid neutralizer—as their only active ingredient. (Examples include *ALternaGEL, Amphojel,* and *Basaljel.*) Such products are recommended only for people who are sensitive to magnesium's laxative effect.

Aluminum hydroxide causes constipation. It's used mainly in combination with magnesium hydroxide, to counteract the latter's laxative effect. Some of the many brands based on this combination include *Aludrox, Delcid, Gelusil, Kolantyl, Maalox, Mylanta,* and *WinGel.* A related magnesium-aluminum compound called magaldrate forms the basis of *Riopan.*

The aluminum-hydroxide/magnesium-hydroxide combinations are the type that physicians most often recommend for long-term, frequent use. Ideally, the constipating and laxative components should balance each other out. But chronic users often experience one or the other problem, more commonly the laxative effect.

Until recently, it was thought that the aluminum in antacids passed harmlessly through the digestive tract without being absorbed into the bloodstream. It's now known that some of the aluminum is absorbed. People with normal kidney function eliminate most of this absorbed aluminum in their urine, but those with impaired kidney function do not. Studies indicate that aluminum can accumulate in certain sites in the body, including the brain and the parathyroid glands. The aluminum-containing antacids constitute a major source of aluminum in the American diet. According to the Federation of American Societies for Experimental Biology, the average daily aluminum intake is about 20 milligrams, compared with the 100 milligrams contained in a single teaspoon of a typical aluminum-containing antacid. The available evidence suggests that elderly people (many of whom have decreased kidney function) and those with kidney disease should use these antacids only on a physician's advice. It's still too early to say whether the aluminum "load" from such antacids may pose a health risk for the general population. Despite frequent speculation, there is no persuasive evidence that intake of aluminum from food, antacids, use of aluminum cookware, or antiperspirants plays any role whatever in causing Alzheimer's disease.

Gaviscon is an aluminum/magnesium product that takes a unique approach. According to the manufacturer, Marion Laboratories, Inc., the antacid ingredients do not neutralize stomach acid; rather, they form a foamy layer that floats atop the stomach contents. When the contents back up, the foamy layer precedes the acid into the esophagus, thus protecting the esophageal tissue from irritation. Several clinicians familiar with *Gaviscon* told CU that the product appears to be effective, though no more so than conventional antacids. And this product is considerably more expensive than the others.

The Simethicone Story Simethicone, a so-called antigas ingredient, is added to certain liquid and tablet antacids, such as *Gelusil, Mylanta II,* and *Silain-Gel*. This is the "plus" in *Maalox Plus* and *Riopan Plus*. Simethicone is also available by itself, in tablets such as *Gas-X* and *Mylicon-80*. But monetary relief for drug makers may well be the only kind of relief that simethicone offers.

In 1973, the FDA advisory panel on antacids concluded there was "inadequate evidence" for simethicone's effectiveness as an "antiflatulent" (antigas remedy). Several months later, the FDA overruled its panel and deemed simethicone effective. The agency's decision was influenced partly by two clinical studies carried out and submitted by Plough, Inc., maker of *Di-Gel*. But that did not end the matter. A later FDA advisory panel, reviewing miscellaneous internal drugs, questioned the effectiveness of all antiflatulents, including simethicone. In its 1982 report, the panel said, in effect: "Let's assume, although proof is scanty, that simethicone really does release bubbles trapped in the stomach or intestine. There's no evidence that these small gas bubbles actually cause the bloating, fullness, and pressure that people attribute to them." So far, the FDA has not acted on this panel's conclusion.

None of CU's medical consultants feel that simethicone does much good. They're joined in this opinion by the two FDA advisory panels and by several authoritative medical publications, including *The Medical Letter*.

Neither simethicone nor any other ingredient is likely to help reduce gas. But certain measures can help prevent the gas from reaching the digestive system in the first place. The major, if not only, source of gas in the stomach is swallowed air. It may help to give up gum-chewing, smoking, and drinking carbonated beverages, to eat more slowly, and to not talk with your mouth full.

Sweeteners Antacids are made more palatable by such ingredients as sucrose, peppermint, wintergreen, mint, orange, and citrus flavor. Some brands still include saccharin, a proven animal carcinogen. The FDA tried to ban this additive, but congressional action allowed it to remain in use. Products that contain saccharin must display a warning on the label.

Sorbitol is also used as a sweetener in many antacids, as well as in some "sugar-free" products such as candy, gum, and dietetic foods. In large amounts—5 or 10 grams—sorbitol can cause intestinal problems, primarily diarrhea. Antacids whose sorbitol content might cause such problems (at high doses) include *ALternaGEL* and the liquid versions of *Gaviscon, Gelusil, Mylanta,* and *Mylanta-II.* With about 600 milligrams of sorbitol per teaspoon, routine amounts of these antacids probably won't cause diarrhea. But one clinical study, using a high-dose regimen of *Mylanta-II* to treat ulcer patients, had to switch two-thirds of the patients to another antacid because of diarrhea. According to CU's medical consultants, *Mylanta-II's* sorbitol dose—28 grams per day in that study— may have been responsible.

RECOMMENDATIONS

Self-medication with antacids should be limited to treating occasional heartburn (no more than once a week). Obviously, many people take antacids far more often. Some keep a bottle of liquid antacid close by and rarely venture out without a roll of tablets. Unfortunately for them, persistent heartburn or upset stomach has become an accepted part of life. It's easy to fall into the antacid habit. *Tums* and *Rolaids,* sweet and minty, are right there on the candy rack next to *Lifesavers* and *Clorets.* *Tums* tablets even come in different flavors. The antacid abuser, however, is merely sugarcoating the stomach problem, often for months or years.

Antacid abuse can aggravate some gastrointestinal problems and mask others that may be serious. For these reasons, persistent heartburn or upset stomach that lasts more than two weeks calls for evaluation by a physician. The cause, if it can be identified, can often be effectively treated.

It is really not possible to say that one brand of antacid will work better than another. Under the FDA's definition of effectiveness, a standard dose of any brand of antacid should help relieve heartburn. Until someone actually compares antacids in a clinical study, the best advice to follow is: Buy the least expensive antacid with the active ingredient(s) you can tolerate and with the taste and form (tablet or liquid) that appeal to you.

Finally, follow these precautions:

- Do not use any antacid regularly for more than two weeks, except with the advice and supervision of a physician.
- Restrict sodium bicarbonate antacids to occasional use only.
- Do not take calcium carbonate antacids for prolonged periods, except in low doses intended for prevention of osteoporosis.
- Give preference to products with magnesium and possibly aluminum ingredients, particularly if antacids must be used for extended periods.
- If you are on a sodium-restricted diet, stick to an antacid low in sodium.

- If you have kidney problems, consult your physician before using any antacid.
- Don't take antacids containing aluminum, calcium, or magnesium at the same time you take a prescription antibiotic that contains tetracycline. Those three ingredients can interact with tetracycline and reduce its absorption into the bloodstream. In general, there should be at least an hour's interval between taking antacids and *any* other medication.
- If you take antacids in tablet form, be sure to chew them thoroughly for maximum effectiveness.
- Rather than accepting antacid use as a way of life, try to eliminate the cause of your heartburn by following the suggestions on pages 46–47.
- And most important, if repeated or painful episodes of indigestion occur, stop self-diagnosis and self-medication and consult your physician.

5

Constipation and Diarrhea

No organ of the body is as misunderstood and fussed over as the digestive tract. It has been purged, irrigated, and massaged, all in the name of an obsessive concern with the daily bowel movement. Many believe that the waste matter left after digestion must be expelled twenty-four to forty-eight hours after the food is eaten. The fallacy of this notion was revealed in an experiment supervised by the late Walter C. Alverez, M.D. A group of healthy young medical students swallowed sets of gelatin capsules containing many small glass beads. Two of the students passed about 85 percent of the beads in twenty-four hours; most took four days to eliminate three-fourths of the beads; some passed only half of the beads in nine days. Those who passed the majority of the beads in twenty-four hours had poorly formed stools containing undigested material. Those with a slower rate usually had well-formed stools showing evidence of good digestion. Some of the participants with the slower rates had believed that they were constipated.

Alverez likened the colon and its fecal contents to a railroad siding on which three freight cars are standing. Every day a new car arrives and bumps the end one off, leaving three again. But occasionally one arrives at the siding with such force that it bumps all three off, and then three days must elapse before the siding is full again. In other words, when the colon is cleaned out by a purge or large bowel movement, nothing more should be expected for several days.

Nor does everyone operate on a once-a-day schedule. It is common to find people in perfect health who defecate two or three times a day, and others who have a single evacuation every two or three days. There are many individuals who have bowel movements at still longer intervals without the slightest ill effect.

Constipation, then, cannot be defined in terms of a daily bowel movement, but must be related to each person's normal functioning. What's more, missing a few bowel movements should cause no alarm. After a few days, things generally return to normal, and the rhythm is reestablished.

Indeed, most cases of constipation cure themselves without intervention. This is fortunate because, commercial advertising to the contrary, there is no such thing as a perfect, natural, or entirely harmless laxative.

A mild laxative can be beneficial in some instances. When, for example, there is temporary difficulty in evacuation due to emotional stress, traveling, or change in diet, there is no harm in taking a mild laxative for a day or two. And in some cases of chronic constipation—if it definitely has been proved to exist and there is no organic cause—a physician may suggest a laxative to help relieve the condition. But the widespread overdependence on laxatives, which supports the sale of more than 700 different over-the-counter (OTC) products, can be explained only by an equally widespread misunderstanding of constipation and the drugs used to treat it.

All types of laxatives have some disadvantages. Moreover, the distinction that the advertisers make between mild laxatives and harsh cathartics is highly deceptive. *Any* material taken by mouth to promote evacuation of the intestine is a cathartic drug; a laxative is simply a mild cathartic. But the strength of a laxative's cathartic effect can vary greatly between people and in the same person at different times.

Laxatives have no doubt contributed to the ills and discomforts of humanity more than the condition they are supposed to relieve. Instances of a ruptured appendix with peritonitis have been recorded in patients who assumed their abdominal pain was caused by constipation and so dosed themselves with laxatives. But constipation is rarely associated with abdominal pain. Nor does the presence of pain mean the bowels need to be cleaned out.

Many people have heard that, at the beginning of a cold or an attack of grippe, flu, or acute tonsillitis, a cathartic should be taken. This myth is a holdover from the Middle Ages when "a dose of the salts" was supposed to cure everything from ague to plague. Yet catharsis does not prevent, cure, or lessen the severity of these or any other illnesses. In acute illness, constipation may simply be associated with dehydration, poor intake of food, or prolonged inactivity. To purge a patient who is already suffering from depleted fluid reserves is foolish—and may even be disastrous.

IRRITABLE BOWEL SYNDROME: ALTERNATING CONSTIPATION AND DIARRHEA

Most often, bowel dysfunction reflects emotional stresses. Such influences on the colon can cause opposing responses in different people—or even in the same individual. In one person they may speed up bowel transit time for ingested foodstuffs and cause diarrhea with occasional mucus in the stool. In another they may slow bowel activity and cause hard, dry, and infrequent stools. In a third they may lead to intestinal spasms perceived as painful abdominal cramps, with alternating periods of diarrhea and constipation.

When these conditions persist or recur, they are known collectively as *irritable bowel syndrome*. This is the likely diagnosis in the case of longstanding bowel complaints associated with worry, fear, and anxiety. The irritable bowel syndrome is a complex disorder probably triggered by many factors, particularly emotional upsets. Irregular peristalsis (the wavelike, propelling contraction of the intestinal tract) results not only in abdominal pains and distention but also in excessive passage of gas; and hard stools often alternate with looser stools. Management of the irritable bowel syndrome consists first of ruling out a definable cause. Careful selection of diet, including an increase of fiber content, can be helpful. Reducing stress through regular exercise and relaxation techniques is important. Professional counseling to treat anxiety or other underlying psychological disorders may be necessary. (Bloody stools, which are not usually associated with the irritable bowel syndrome, always require consultation with a physician.)

The irritable bowel syndrome is no longer considered the only cause for complaints of bloating, gaseous distention, and intermittent loose stools. It has been shown that for some people a more likely explanation may be what formerly was called an intestinal "allergy." A physician may discover through careful questioning that the discomfort is due to a food intolerance. (See page 41 for a discussion of food allergy and food intolerance.) A frequent cause is the lack of an intestinal enzyme—lactase— which is essential for the proper digestion of milk products. These foods tend to precipitate episodes of abdominal discomfort. The ingestion of certain other foods can cause similar patterns such as florid diarrhea, experienced by patients with nontropical sprue and celiac disease—an intestinal malfunction caused by intolerance to gluten (the insoluble protein constituent of wheat and other grains).

Unfortunately, the symptoms of an irritable bowel are not always evident. For example, the emotional factors responsible for bowel dysfunction may not be obvious, so that sufferers may not be able to know that their constipation or diarrhea is of this type. This is another reason why proper diagnosis is important before a course of treatment for chronic constipation or diarrhea is begun.

CAUSES AND TREATMENT OF DIARRHEA

The affliction commonly referred to as "acute gastroenteritis" usually involves two or three days of diarrhea, along with fever and general malaise. It is thought to be viral in origin. Healthy individuals are able to withstand such illness with only minor discomfort. The very young and the very old, regardless of their health, fare less well. Because they are especially sensitive to the need for adequate fluid replacement, some may even require hospitalization.

Most attacks of diarrhea tend to be self-limited, with the symptoms relieved (with or without medication) in a few days. However, diarrhea can be protracted, lasting more than a week. In the beginning stages, underlying causes of protracted diarrhea—such as giardiasis, amebic dysentery, Crohn's disease, or ulcerative colitis—may be difficult to diagnose. Because specific therapy for such diseases must often await diagnosis, it is important during a prolonged bout of diarrhea to have microscopic and bacteriological examinations made of the stool, as well as a sigmoidoscopic examination of the rectum, in which a physician may directly observe the rectum and lower bowel through a flexible, lighted tube called a sigmoidoscope. X rays of the bowel also may be necessary.

If an attack of diarrhea does not subside in a day or so, or if diarrhea is accompanied at any time by fever, severe abdominal pain, or bloody stools, don't self-medicate. Consult a physician. In any case, a person suffering from diarrhea should drink plenty of liquids to offset loss of fluids in the watery stools. Decreasing the amount of roughage (or bulk producers) in the diet—for example, cutting out most raw fruits and raw vege-tables—and following the time-honored treatment of rice and bananas may reduce the severity of the attack.

OTC preparations commonly used for acute diarrhea, such as kaolin/pectin mixtures (*Kaodene* and *Kaopectate,* among others), are less effec-tive than antidiarrheal drugs containing narcotics, which require a pre-scription in most states. Physicians may prescribe diphenoxylate (Lom-otil) or loperamide (Imodium). (*Imodium* in liquid form is now available OTC; capsules are still available only by prescription.) These two drugs provide relatively prompt relief from diarrhea. In the amounts used for occasional diarrheal attacks, they should present no problem of dependency.

The use of diphenoxylate and loperamide is inadvisable for infants and young children. Toxicity has been observed with minimal dosage. Nor have they been proved safe for use by pregnant women. And they should be used with caution, if at all, in acute infectious diarrhea, since some experts believe these medications can actually prolong the disease.

Some medications frequently cause loose, watery bowel movements. The most common offenders include such antibiotics as erythromycin, ampicillin, and tetracycline. Also capable of provoking diarrhea are some magnesium-containing antacids (see page 51) and large doses of ascorbic acid (vitamin C).

CAUSES AND TREATMENTS OF CONSTIPATION

When true chronic constipation is present, it may result from overem-phasis on toilet training in childhood, crowded living conditions, poor diet, or similar behavioral factors. Something as simple as improper toilet habits is frequently an underlying cause. When the urge to defecate is dis-regarded, the sensation passes. It usually returns again during the day, especially after a meal, but if the call is consistently disobeyed day after day, the rectum may eventually fail to signal the need for evacuation. The result may be severe constipation.

Why is the call disregarded? It may be suppressed, or it may be over-whelmed by other and stronger stimuli, similar to loss of one's appetite on hearing bad news. It also may be neglected because of the pressure of school or work, or perhaps because there is a morning train to catch, or only one bathroom for a large family.

Many commonly used OTC and prescription drugs are also apt to cause constipation. Antacids may often be a source of difficulty (see Chapter 4). Among prescription drugs the most notorious offenders are narcotics such as codeine, opium, and oxycodone (the active ingredient in Percocet and Percodan). Another class of compounds capable of causing constipation includes those affecting the parasympathetic nervous system. Among these drugs are gastrointestinal antispasmodics such as propantheline (Pro-Banthine), antidepressants such as imipramine (Tofranil), and major tranquilizers such as chlorpromazine (Thorazine). Should constipation become a severe side effect, a physician may decrease dosage or switch to another medication.

The misuse of laxatives is another important cause of chronic constipation. Whatever the original reason for using a laxative, repeated purging in time brings changes in the lining and muscle tone of the bowel; the lining can become irritated and inflamed, and with long-continued catharsis muscular reflexes can become so diminished that stronger and stronger stimulation is required to produce activity. Chronic laxative abusers may also unknowingly be depleting their body of potassium, resulting in muscle weakness. Moreover, few users of cathartics have not suffered from fissure of the anus or hemorrhoids. Such ailments often make defecation so painful that the sufferer tends to postpone a visit to the toilet, with the same results as those occurring in a person who is too busy. (Hemorrhoids, discussed in Chapter 6, may also be caused by chronic constipation or diarrhea.)

A small percentage of patients with constipation may have an organic disease such as diverticulitis or cancer. This cause is most likely to be found in adults who previously have had regular and satisfactory evacuation but then begin to experience a persistent change in the character or frequency of bowel movements. To investigate the possibility of organic disease, a physician may directly observe the rectum and lower bowel through a sigmoidoscope. The physician also may have a radiologist perform a barium-enema X-ray examination to inspect the remainder of the lower bowel. But, to repeat, constipation is not commonly caused by an organic disease. And in general, if constipation has been present for a number of years, the condition probably is not due to disease.

Safe and Effective Laxatives

The Food and Drug Administration (FDA) advisory panel that reviewed OTC laxatives in 1975 judged that 25 percent of the 81 laxative ingredients submitted for review were unsafe or ineffective. Another 20 percent needed further study.

Most of the unsafe and ineffective ingredients are no longer included in the products currently on the market—but, as of this writing, some of the dubious ones are still around. Ingredients judged by the panel to lack "medical or scientific rationale" included vitamins and minerals (as in *Geriplex-FS*) and capsicum (no longer widely marketed as a laxative). The panel recommended that labels list not only the quantity of each active ingredient in a standard dose but also all inactive ingredients as well. It recommended that ingredients judged unsafe or ineffective or lacking in medical or scientific rationale be eliminated from OTC laxative products.

CU's medical consultants suggest that you avoid laxatives containing ingredients that act as bowel stimulants, unless advised by a physician. These drugs include phenolphthalein (*Alophen, Correctol, Espotabs, Evac-Q-Kwik, Evac-U-Gen, Ex-Lax, Feen-A-Mint Pills,* and *Laxcaps*), senna (*Gentlax, Senokot*), bisacodyl (*Carter's Little Pills, Dulcolax*), and cascara (*Nature's Remedy*). All these agents stimulate peristalsis; all can cause severe painful cramping. The FDA panel recommended that stimulant laxatives be labeled with this warning: "Prolonged or continued use of this product can lead to laxative dependency and loss of normal bowel function. Serious side effects from prolonged use or overuse may occur."

Another class of laxatives that increases peristalsis includes saline (salt) cathartics. The most popular salts used are magnesium citrate (citrate of magnesia), magnesium hydroxide (milk of magnesia), and sodium phosphate (*Fleet Phospho-Soda, Sodium Phosphates Oral Solution USP*). Results with these laxatives can be dramatic, depending on the dose used. People with chronic kidney disease, who may have difficulty in excreting magnesium, should be wary about using milk of magnesia. People on salt-restricted diets should avoid laxatives containing sodium.

If you must resort to a laxative, CU's medical consultants recommend that you restrict yourself to a bulk-producing laxative or possibly a stool softener. According to the FDA panel report, "Bulk-forming laxatives are among the safest of laxatives." Bulk-producing laxatives, such as psyllium (*Effer-Syllium, Fiberall, Hydrocil Instant, Konsyl, L.A. Formula,* and *Metamucil*), tend to cause fewer unpleasant side effects than bowel stimulants. Those on salt-restricted diets should note that *Effer-Syllium* and *Metamucil Instant Mix* (both regular and orange flavor) contain a considerable quantity of sodium. (Most bulk producers should be taken with a full glass of water to guard against the remote possibility of intestinal obstruction.)

Synthetic cellulose derivatives—methylcellulose and carboxymethyl cellulose sodium—are sometimes used as bulk-forming laxatives, but usually in combination with other active ingredients. Generic versions of these products are also available.

Stool softeners work for some people, but not for all. These detergent products help fluids to penetrate the stool and increase its water content. Docusate sodium (or calcium) sulfosuccinate is the main detergent or softener, and is marketed under such brand names as *Afko-Lube, Colace, Coloctyl, Comfolax,* docusate sodium, *DioMedicone, Dio-Sul, Disonate, Doxinate, Modane Soft, Regutol,* and *Surfac.*

The brand names on these pages by no means exhaust the list of laxatives on the market. In addition to the preparations based on a single active ingredient, there is a predictably large contingent of combination-type laxatives. Shoppers may find products combining a stool softener with a bulk laxative, or a bowel stimulant with an emollient. Although the FDA panel would allow some products with two active laxative ingredients (but no more than two) to remain on the market, the panel agrees that a single-ingredient product is safest. As always, consumers are urged to read the label carefully.

The laxative market is swamped with label claims that, in the panel's opinion, should be changed. A laxative label should not make assertions about general benefits for good health, regularity, or the relief of indigestion, headaches, or "excessive belching." Instead, it should identify the product as a laxative for the "short-term relief of constipation." Nor should the label warn against the hazards of constipation, because such warnings are "unproven and thus unacceptable," according to the panel.

Also forbidden would be any suggestion that taking a laxative is somehow natural. The panel points out that taking a laxative is never natural. And the label should not suggest that the laxative is particularly appropriate for individuals of a certain sex or age.

Mineral oil (an emollient) has had many loyal fans, particularly among older people. However, use of mineral oil over time—especially by the elderly or disabled—may lead to lipid pneumonia, a chronic lung condition caused by inadvertent inhalation of oil into the lungs. Because of this and other disadvantages, such as rectal leakage and interference with the body's absorption of vitamins A, D, E, and K, mineral oil is no longer a laxative of choice. The drawbacks of mineral oil, however, can be minimized by taking it only occasionally in the smallest effective dosage (about one tablespoon for an adult) on an empty stomach and by not lying down for at least half an hour after ingestion. Because the absorption of mineral oil can be facilitated by docusate sodium, these two agents should not be used at the same time.

Yogurt and acidophilus milk were once in vogue for the treatment of bowel disorders, including constipation. The nutritive value of yogurt and other fermented milks is essentially the same as that of the whole milk from which they are made; hence they are good foods. And they can be safely consumed by people who have an intolerance to lactose. But, although fermented milks have occasionally been reported to be successful in the treatment of mild constipation, they usually are not of much value. Nor is there any evidence to support the routine use of vitamin B_1, vitamin B_6, or any other vitamin in the treatment of habitual constipation.

Some people may find it more natural, if not as convenient, to use an enema instead of a laxative. As authorities have been saying for many years, it does seem unreasonable to upset 25 feet of intestine with a cathartic when the trouble is in the last 8 inches—the rectum and the anal canal. An enema consisting of a pint of tepid tap water is generally sufficient. While they are relatively expensive, prepackaged disposable enemas (for example, *Fleet*) can be a convenience. But too frequent use of enemas—even once a week, for some people—can result in an inability to initiate a bowel movement without an enema. (High colonic enemas, incidentally, are an antiquated, useless, and sometimes harmful procedure.

They do not cure habitual constipation or remove "toxins," and they certainly do not in any way promote health or prolong life.)

Glycerin and bisacodyl *(Dulcolax)* suppositories have also been employed to stimulate evacuation of the rectum without disturbing the rest of the bowel. Their occasional use does no harm, but most physicians believe that frequent use of suppositories can cause irritation both of the anus and of the mucous membrane of the rectum.

Recommended Treatment of Constipation

Against this background, some rational approaches to the treatment of constipation become clear. For temporary constipation, the obvious thing to do is nothing; let nature take its course, and the condition will resolve itself. If you have been taking laxatives for constipation, the first thing to do is to stop taking them. Many people who have done so at the insistence of a physician have been surprised to find that, after a few days or a week, the bowels begin to move effectively again.

You might find it helpful to add fiber, or roughage, to your diet in the form of fruits, vegetables, breads, and whole-grain cereals. Fiber resists digestion and reaches the large intestine virtually unchanged. There, it speeds the passage of feces through the intestine, lessening the strain of a bowel movement. Fiber also retains water and adds to the bulk, softness, and weight of stool—all factors in easing strain. (Adding liquids to the diet contributes to the softening effect.)

Remember, however, that each person's digestive system works differently. Some people can eat a high percentage of fiber without the slightest inconvenience. The same meal can cause others distress. If such a diet causes pain, distention, mucus in the stool, or other evidence of irritation, a physician should be consulted. (See Chapter 11 for other recommendations regarding fiber consumption.)

Among the more valuable foods for fiber are bran, spinach, raw carrots, and whole fruit. Bran, often promoted for the relief of constipation, may be useful particularly to those who do not object to swift and dramatic results. Cereals with the highest bran content include *Fiber One* and Kellogg's *All-Bran* and *All-Bran with Extra Fiber.* Prunes, the traditional friend of the constipated, provide bulk and contain a chemical that stimulates peristalsis. Peristalsis may also be aided through use of prune extract or prune juice.

The role of exercise in the treatment of constipation has been promoted by many. It may divert one's thoughts from work or household worries, conferring a sense of relaxation that facilitates a bowel movement. Massaging the abdominal muscles is a waste of time as therapy for constipation. And the value of drinking large quantities of water—even hot water flavored with lemon—has been highly overrated. However, any of these measures may have an important psychological effect.

As stated previously, on certain occasions, a mild laxative for a day or two may help you to overcome a temporary disruption caused by stress, travel, or diet. Your best choice is the mildest laxative that produces results—usually a bulk producer or perhaps a stool softener.

Some people complain of headache or sluggishness, or they just plain worry if they don't have a regular bowel movement; for such people it may be less harmful to use a laxative once in a while than to fret.

If simple measures don't clear up constipation within a week or so, the problem requires advice from a physician. Rational treatment must be based on the cause, and that can be established only through physical examination, careful questioning, and perhaps testing. Daily living habits and diet must be taken into account. Often a laxative is prescribed, as a temporary measure, to promote evacuation while the patient tries to reestablish a normal bowel routine. The laxative may then be gradually withdrawn.

Constipation in children requires special consideration. In the majority of cases it is due to oversolicitous attitudes on the part of parents. When a child senses anxiety in a parent about bowel function, the child too may become tense and unable to relax, and relaxation is essential to a normal bowel movement.

If constipation develops in a child, what should be done? A good rule to follow in treating a child's constipation is "Don't." A child will not become ill from a temporary lapse, and in a day or two normal bowel activity usually reestablishes itself spontaneously. If constipation is due to an acute ailment, medical care for the illness—not a laxative—is required. If constipation tends to recur, it may be due to improper diet or bowel habits, and a physician should be consulted. The prohibition of

laxatives, suppositories, and enemas for children with constipation cannot be too strongly emphasized.

Pregnant women are especially susceptible to constipation because of
the direct pressure of the enlarged uterus on the rectum as well as the
relaxing effect of elevated hormone levels on the muscles of the bowel.
But a pregnant woman should not routinely take laxatives—or any medication—without consulting a physician. There's no harm, however, in
adding some roughage to the diet.

Help for Hemorrhoids?

Hemorrhoids bother about half of all Americans at some time in their lives, usually after age 30. Many others have hemorrhoids without even realizing it. One recent study showed that, of 241 healthy people reporting for physical exams, 82 percent had hemorrhoids.

Hemorrhoids are essentially swollen blood vessels in the anal canal and lower rectum. These vessels bulge inward and narrow the anorectal passage. Hemorrhoid sufferers may experience bleeding during bowel movements, itching in the anal area, and a feeling of lingering fullness in the rectum after a bowel movement. Occasionally, hemorrhoids also cause outright pain.

There are two types of hemorrhoids, internal and external.

INTERNAL HEMORRHOIDS

Most experts now regard internal hemorrhoids as normal anatomic structures. They result when the "cushions" of blood vessels and connective tissue that line the lower rectum and anal canal become swollen and protrude from the rectal wall. The cushions gradually become elongated and descend toward the anus. There are three main cushions, which is why the typical case of internal hemorrhoids involves three hemorrhoids.

What transforms the cushions into hemorrhoids? Aging seems to be one factor. The connective-tissue fibers that anchor the cushions to the rectal wall become looser and weaker as people age. That may explain why hemorrhoids are quite rare in childhood. Perhaps more important, however, are the forces that propel the cushions downward toward the anus. Most authorities believe that chronic constipation (see Chapter 5) is the main cause of hemorrhoids. Over time, as constipated people strain to evacuate their bowels, the increased pressure in the rectum causes blood vessels in the cushions to become chronically engorged with blood. That gradually distends and weakens the vessel walls. The hemorrhoids then tend to bleed easily as passing feces buffet the stretched and fragile mucous-membrane covering.

Pressure from the frequent bowel movements associated with diarrhea (see Chapter 5) can also cause hemorrhoids. Indeed, any prolonged period on the toilet focuses considerable pressure on the anal area—even if all you do there is read.

Hemorrhoids are also encouraged by other factors that create chronic increased abdominal pressure. They're common during pregnancy, for example, and among people who exert themselves strenuously at work or who stand in one place for long periods. Additional factors contributing to hemorrhoids include heredity (hemorrhoids tend to run in families), low daily intake of liquids, and faulty bowel function due to overuse of laxatives and enemas.

The most common symptom of internal hemorrhoids—and often the only one in mild cases—is bleeding, apparent from bright red blood on the toilet paper or coating the feces. (*Hemorrhoid* comes from the Greek words *haema,* "blood," and *rhoe,* "flow.") Bleeding often occurs intermittently, with weeks or months between episodes. As the downward pressures exerted on internal hemorrhoids stretch them toward the anus, the sufferer may also experience a feeling of incomplete evacuation following a bowel movement.

On wiping, you can feel a hemorrhoid as a lump that gradually recedes into the rectum by itself or can be gently eased back in with a finger. (*Piles,* from the Latin word for ball, is another term for hemorrhoids.) In severe cases, an internal hemorrhoid projects from the anus and can't be pushed back. This "completely prolapsed hemorrhoid" can be quite painful.

In most cases, however, internal hemorrhoids are not painful, since their mucous-membrane covering has no nerve endings to sense pain. As anyone who has seen ads for hemorrhoid remedies knows, internal hemorrhoids often cause irritation, itching, and burning. Those symptoms are generally caused by mucus and feces that adhere to the bulging hemorrhoid and irritate the skin around the anal opening.

EXTERNAL HEMORRHOIDS

External hemorrhoids are another story. These arise from swollen clumps of blood vessels located around the rim of the anus or just inside. External hemorrhoids are not covered by nerveless mucous membrane but by one of the body's most sensitive areas, the skin in and around the anus. When a small blood clot forms in one of the swollen blood vessels, it stretches this sensitive skin and brings on sudden and often severe pain. Such a hemorrhoid "attack," which usually results from strenuous physical exertion, is known as a thrombosed external hemorrhoid. It can be felt with a finger as a firm, tender, rounded mass about the size of a pea. The pain lasts until the clot softens—usually in a few days, with or without the use of hemorrhoid remedies. In very painful cases, a doctor can provide almost immediate relief by making a small incision and releasing the clot.

MISDIAGNOSIS

Often, symptoms that people attribute to hemorrhoids are not a result of hemorrhoids at all. Itching may be caused by poor anal hygiene, perianal warts, intestinal worms, overgrowth of fungi from use of antibiotics, psoriasis, nervous scratching, and many other causes. Pain can result from fissures (small cracks in the skin surrounding the anus) or from infections in the anal area.

But the most serious misdiagnoses involve bleeding, the most common symptom of hemorrhoids. For instance, bleeding can be a symptom of colorectal cancer—a disease that kills more than 50,000 Americans each year. Persistent or recurrent bleeding demands medical attention. Unfortunately, many people tend to ignore rectal bleeding—either out of embarrassment about being examined or out of fear of discovering they have cancer. Chances are, hemorrhoids are responsible. But you owe it to yourself to rule out other causes. That requires investigations that may include barium X-ray studies or the use of instruments (the sigmoidoscope or colonoscope) to examine the wall of the bowel. Once more serious conditions have been ruled out, various treatments can help alleviate hemorrhoid symptoms.

PREVENTION AND SELF-TREATMENT

There are two major steps people can take on their own to minimize the symptoms of hemorrhoids. One is to increase the amount of fiber in the diet—a step that may also help prevent hemorrhoids from developing. Since straining on the toilet due to constipation is probably the main cause of hemorrhoids, it follows that avoiding constipation is an important part of prevention and, in mild cases, cure. Adding fiber to the diet is the only treatment necessary for about half of all cases of hemorrhoids. (High-fiber diet and other ways to avoid or resolve constipation are discussed in Chapter 5, page 65.)

The other way to minimize symptoms is to practice good anal care. Hygienic habits can help control irritation and itching, whether caused by hemorrhoids or not. Most important is to keep the skin around the anus clean and dry. Residual fecal matter keeps the area moist and can irritate the skin. But vigorous wiping with dry toilet paper may make things worse. Instead, swab the area after each bowel movement using toilet paper moistened with warm water. Then gently pat the area dry. For convenience and a soothing effect, some people like premoistened wipes such as *Gentz Wipes, Mediconet, Preparation H Cleansing Pads, Rantex,* or *Tucks Pads.*

Soap residues can irritate, so always rinse off completely after showering or bathing. If soaps do cause irritation, you can clean the anal area with a product like *Balneol* perianal cleansing lotion.

A sitz bath—sitting in warm tap water a few inches deep for 10 to 15 minutes—is a time-honored treatment for anal discomfort. Three or four sitz baths per day for a few days may provide considerable relief. A bathtub works fine, or you can buy a portable plastic sitz bath that fits over the toilet.

Since perspiration can irritate the anal area, avoid tight undergarments and pantyhose. Loose cotton underwear is best. A light sprinkling of talcum powder in the area can help absorb moisture.

Drugstore Remedies

Before seeking professional care, most hemorrhoid sufferers try to treat themselves—typically for a year or longer—with over-the-counter (OTC) remedies. By far the biggest seller is *Preparation H*. According to industry sources in 1986, this product alone accounts for more than half the $200 million Americans spend yearly in search of relief at the drug counter. Next in line are *Anusol, Tronolane, Nupercainal,* and others.

CU's medical consultants have reservations about the use of some of the leading OTC remedies. They contain a number of ingredients, including anesthetics, astringents, counterirritants, and skin protectants. Some of these ingredients can trigger an allergic reaction and make irritation worse. Peruvian balsam, an astringent used in *Anusol* ointment and other products, caused allergic reactions in 10 to 20 percent of patients tested with it.

The worst offenders are the "caine" anesthetics—benzocaine, dibucaine, and others. These chemically similar anesthetics are notorious for causing allergic skin reactions. CU's medical consultants recommend against products containing them, including *Americaine, BiCozene, Lanacane, Nupercainal,* and *Medicone.* Another anesthetic, pramoxine hydrochloride, differs chemically from the "caine" anesthetics and appears to cause fewer allergic problems. It is found in *Tronolane* and other products.

Despite their diverse composition, most hemorrhoid remedies make the same basic claim—temporary relief of pain and itching. But *Preparation H* is famous for an additional claim—relief of swelling. Any bland cream or ointment, even without active ingredients, can soothe irritated skin. *Preparation H* can probably do that job as well as its competitors. But none has been proved to shrink swollen hemorrhoids. *The Medical Letter,* a respected newsletter for physicians, concluded back in 1975: "There is no acceptable evidence that the heavily promoted *Preparation H* . . . can shrink hemorrhoids, reduce inflammation, or heal injured tissue."

Hemorrhoid products are marketed in three basic forms—cleansers, suppositories, and creams or ointments.

Cleansers   The best hemorrhoid products, we believe, help keep the anal area clean. They include *Preparation H Cleansing Pads* and *Tucks Pads.*

Suppositories   It makes little sense to use hemorrhoid suppositories. After a suppository is inserted into the anus, it often slides up into the upper rectum, bypassing the spot that needs treatment. True, a suppository can lubricate the rectum, and thus make hard bowel movements less painful. But any effect on the hemorrhoids themselves is minimal at best. Many of the suppository products are also available as creams or ointments.

Creams and Ointments   These may help soothe irritation. Creams are generally preferable to ointments. Ointments, which are greasier, tend to retain moisture, which may encourage itching and irritation in the anal area. Hydrocortisone, present in several products, is an effective anti-itch ingredient. But its overuse may lead to dependency and can cause thinning of the skin, which results in more fissures and bleeding.

Self-treatment with hemorrhoid remedies may aggravate the trouble and sensitize the skin. But even worse, it can cause serious conditions to be overlooked. Persistent or recurring itching, pain, or bleeding in the anorectal area should not be ignored or treated in a casual fashion with OTC remedies. Each of these symptoms should be evaluated by a physician and treated appropriately.

PROFESSIONAL TREATMENT

If hemorrhoid symptoms persist despite self-treatment, you might want to seek professional treatment. Three relatively painless office procedures can ease most cases of internal hemorrhoids and may prevent them from worsening to the point where surgery is necessary. The procedures—injection, rubber-banding, and photocoagulation—relieve symptoms mainly by shrinking hemorrhoids somewhat and anchoring them in place.

Injection   To shrink the hemorrhoid and its blood vessels, the physician injects a liquid into the mucous membrane near the hemorrhoid. This technique works well for treating small bleeding hemorrhoids that haven't yet protruded into the anal canal. It is also useful for treating hemorrhoids that protrude through the anus during defecation and then retract. Repeat treatments every two or three years may be necessary.

Rubber-banding   This technique, the most widely used office treatment, is mainly for hemorrhoids that protrude on defecation and retract spontaneously or are easily pushed back in. A special instrument fits a small rubber band over part of the hemorrhoid. The tight rubber band stops the blood flow to the pinched-off portion, which falls off in about a week. This procedure often causes some discomfort until the end result is achieved.

Photocoagulation In this recently developed technique, a device called a photocoagulator focuses infrared light into a fine point at the end of a probe, which in effect spot-welds the hemorrhoid in place. Photocoagulation can often substitute for either of the other office procedures, and recent studies indicate that it may be the fastest and least painful of the three.

Surgical Treatment

Hemorrhoids that reach the painful point where they protrude from the anus and can't be pushed in may have to be removed surgically. The surgical procedure, called a *hemorrhoidectomy*, is performed less often now than it was 20 years ago, mainly because the newer office treatments described above often suffice.

A modern hemorrhoidectomy is much less painful than it once was. Previously, the operation was always done under general anesthesia. It required a week in the hospital and two to three weeks of recovery at home. Now local anesthesia is often used; many patients return home the day after surgery and go back to work after a few days of rest. Some doctors perform the operation on an outpatient basis.

Lately, some surgeons have begun to use a new and controversial operation, the laser hemorrhoidectomy. Proponents claim it is less painful than the traditional operation and removes hemorrhoids more completely; critics contend it is no better than traditional surgery. The verdict will have to await clinical trials.

Insomnia

If you frequently find yourself staring at the bedroom ceiling at 3 A.M., you're not alone. Millions of Americans have trouble falling asleep or staying asleep.

Everyone suffers an occasional restless night. Too much caffeine or an upset stomach may steal a few hours. But frequent insomnia often has less obvious causes, and effective therapy can be elusive. Some commonly used remedies, such as alcohol and over-the-counter (OTC) drugs, may even complicate the problem.

Common though it is, not everyone who complains of insomnia actually suffers from it. Studies in sleep-research laboratories reveal that many people sleep more than they think they do. Researchers estimate that at least one-third of all people who consider themselves insomniacs get as much sleep as people who consider themselves normal sleepers.

Some people believe they're missing out if they sleep less than seven or eight hours. But the need for sleep varies widely from person to person, commonly ranging from as little as four hours to as much as 10. Even missing most of a night's sleep once in a while is unlikely to have any serious effect—except for the worry about getting through the next day.

Many older people find that they just can't sleep as they used to. Sometimes, that's because daytime naps interfere with a full night's sleep. Other causes include the need for frequent urination due to an enlarged prostate gland, or shortness of breath and cough arising from heart or lung disease. What's more, the quality of sleep itself changes with age. Older people tend to spend more time in light sleep. Their sleep is often more fitful and punctuated by frequent awakenings. These normal changes in sleep patterns and physical problems that occur with aging are responsible for much of what's perceived as insomnia.

THREE FORMS OF INSOMNIA

For the millions who are plagued by insomnia, an understanding of the different forms can be the first step toward a good night's sleep. What helps in some types of insomnia can be useless or even counterproductive in others.

Sleep-research specialists commonly sort insomnia into one of three types: *transient, short-term,* or *chronic.* Transient describes occasional episodes of insomnia among normal sleepers, who may endure a few restless nights because of jet lag, a fight with the boss, a new romance, or any one of countless anxiety-provoking or exciting prospects.

Short-term insomnia, which may last up to a few weeks, generally arises from temporary, stressful situations. It's usually associated with the death of a loved one, job loss, fear of having a serious illness, and similar experiences.

Chronic insomnia, on the other hand, may go on for months or years, many times with no obvious explanation. In some people, it may be a result of organic illness or a symptom of an underlying psychiatric problem, such as depression. In others, it may occur in association with chronic use of sleep medication, excessive alcohol intake, or "biological clock" disturbances from shift work or jet lag. Disorders characterized by involuntary jerking or "restless" leg movements can lead to chronic insomnia. Recently, disorders of the upper airway (nasal passage, back of the mouth, and upper windpipe) have also received much attention as possible causes.

Worry about insomnia can create a self-fulfilling prophecy. After a few nights of sleeplessness, some people panic—and, as a result, are even less likely to sleep well the next night. The distress that they feel when they can't sleep may then become associated with the bedroom itself. When they go to bed, they become aroused rather than sleepy.

Various drugs can also promote—and sustain—insomnia. Stimulants like caffeine and appetite suppressants are well-known offenders. Betablockers (atenolol, nadolol, propranolol, and others) used for hypertension can cause disturbing dreams and subsequent wakefulness. Even some drugs prescribed for insomnia can interfere with normal sleep patterns and perpetuate the condition.

With all these possibilities to consider, intensive investigation is sometimes necessary to identify and solve the underlying cause of chronic insomnia. This may require a visit to your physician or even to a sleep clinic—a center that specializes in the diagnosis and treatment of sleep disorders. Before you call in the medical cavalry, though, there are some steps you can try yourself.

SLEEP HYGIENE

Any number of common practices can interfere with a good night's sleep. Accordingly, sleep-disorder specialists advise the following "sleep hygiene" measures to counter sleep-robbing habits:

- Establish a fixed sleep schedule. Go to bed and get up at set times, and don't try to make up for lost sleep on weekends or holidays. Eat at the same time each day.
- Don't nap, day or evening.
- Never stay in bed when you can't sleep. Instead of tossing and turning, force yourself to get up and go to another room. Do something you find relaxing—read, listen to music, watch television—until you're sleepy.
- Exercise regularly, preferably in the morning or well before dinner.
- Avoid caffeine-containing tea, coffee, and soft drinks for at least four hours before bedtime. Also avoid OTC diet pills, since these products may contain phenylpropanolamine (PPA), a stimulant that also doubles as a decongestant (see page 25).
- Try to plan evening activities that are conducive to relaxation, including light exercise such as a leisurely walk. Sexual activity can also be an effective soporific for some people.
- Minimize external distractions that may disturb you at bedtime. For example, use dark window shades or eye coverings to block out annoying light, or soundproof your room to reduce noise.

DRAWBACKS OF SELF-MEDICATION

Some people find an occasional nightcap or nonprescription sleep aid helpful for inducing drowsiness. But when used repeatedly, say sleep-disorder specialists, such self-prescribed remedies are either ineffectual or counterproductive.

Alcohol is the most commonly used nonprescription drug for insomnia. While it may help at first, it can disrupt your sleep patterns over time. Within a few weeks, moreover, the user usually begins to develop a tolerance to alcohol, and increasingly larger amounts may be needed to produce the same effect. This can lead to a vicious cycle in which an insomniac drinks more and more alcohol, in turn disrupting sleep further.

The active ingredients in OTC sleep aids are antihistamines, which were originally developed to treat allergies—still their primary function. One side effect of antihistamines is drowsiness—often a bane to allergy sufferers. Ever resourceful, drug companies have salvaged this unwanted side effect as a remedy for insomnia.

Antihistamines with the greatest sedative effect are diphenhydramine (found in *Nytol, Sleep-Eze 3, Sominex 2,* and others) and doxylamine *(Unisom).* Pyrilamine *(Quiet World* and others) generally produces less drowsiness and more stomach upset. However, individual response to antihistamines varies greatly; in fact, some people—usually children but occasionally elderly people—become aroused rather than drowsy.

Diphenhydramine is also an effective cough suppressant. Such a triple-threat (to allergy, cough, and insomnia) drug conceivably might serve one possible use: If you can't sleep because of allergy woes and a hacking cough, a product such as *Nytol* might do the trick. So, too, might any remedy containing diphenhydramine.

On the other hand, if you suffer from insomnia, we do not recommend OTC sleep aids. If you really need a medication—and you may not—you should take the most effective one.

PRESCRIPTION DRUGS

If insomnia persists despite sleep-hygiene measures, it's time for professional help, especially if the problem is disrupting your life. An internist or other primary-care physician is a good first choice.

If the visit is brief, and you find yourself with a quick prescription for sleep medication, you may not be getting the help you need. A responsible physician, especially when helping a new patient, will spend time taking a thorough medical and sleep history, including questions about your physical health, "restless legs" syndrome, sleepiness during the daytime, medications you take, and other possible clues. Depending on the problem, your doctor may conduct a full-scale medical exam, prescribe a short course of medication, or refer you to a sleep clinic.

The most accepted use of prescription sleeping pills is for episodes of transient or short-term insomnia—during a hospitalization, for example, or after a death in the family. Where barbiturates—phenobarbital, secobarbital (Seconal), and others—were once commonly prescribed, benzodiazepines are now the drugs of choice due to their relative safety and efficacy. Benzodiazepines are the family of tranquilizers and sleep-inducing agents that includes chlordiazepoxide (Librium), diazepam (Valium), flurazepam (Dalmane), temazepam (Restoril), and triazolam (Halcion). The choice usually depends on the properties of the drug and the patient's needs, such as whether a long-acting or short-acting agent is preferable. All but Halcion are available generically.

Like alcohol, these drugs interfere with normal sleep patterns by suppressing the dreaming stage of sleep. Discontinuing long-term use can result in a "rebound" of dreaming, including an increase in nightmares typical of alcohol withdrawal. Also as with alcohol, tolerance to the drugs develops over time, with increasing doses required to achieve the same effect. Accordingly, most sleep specialists recommend that the drugs be used in insomnia only for limited periods, such as a few weeks. Some doctors advise their patients to take the medication every other night. The common guideline is "the smallest effective dose for the shortest time necessary."

In short, drugs are not ideal for treating chronic insomnia. Although they are still used in some instances, the trend in sleep-disorder therapy has been to develop other strategies for relieving long-term problems.

OTHER PATHS TO SLEEP

Sometimes, more hours spent in bed can mean less time sleeping. Hoping to make up for lost sleep, an insomniac may go to bed at 10 P.M. and stay there doggedly until 8 A.M. But much of the time may be spent in brief dozing and repeated awakenings. The result is a scant four or five hours of sleep for 10 hours of concerted effort.

To break that cycle, psychologist Arthur Spielman, director of the Sleep Disorders Center at the City College of New York, devised a technique called "sleep restriction." A person who ekes out only five hours of sleep is allowed only five hours in bed; a four-hour sleeper, just four hours. In this approach, the patient typically goes to bed several hours later than usual but arises the same time each morning, sleepy or not.

Daytime naps are prohibited, even if the person has to move about repeatedly to stay awake. If the quality of sleep improves—fewer awakenings, for example—the time in bed is gradually extended until the patient achieves the amount of sleep desired. Early studies indicate that the method can be effective.

When a person's problem involves an inability to fall asleep until early morning hours, an approach called "chronotherapy" may be used. It gradually adjusts the hours of bedtime and arising until the desired sleep time is achieved.

As a sleep strategy, nutritional tactics may seem least worrisome, though not necessarily most effective. For years, studies have suggested that L-tryptophan, a naturally occurring amino acid in food, may help to promote sleep. Foods high in carbohydrates, such as cereal or crackers, increase the level of L-tryptophan in the blood. Protein-rich foods tend to decrease it. L-tryptophan is also marketed in pill form, at up to $15 a bottle in some health-food stores. Many sleep specialists keep an open mind about L-tryptophan, but few suspect it will ever play more than an ancillary role in relieving insomnia. There's no harm in trying some cookies, a bowl of cereal, or a glass of warm milk. When L-tryptophan is taken in supplement form, though, large doses initially tend to produce nausea. Doses low enough to be tolerated seem to work best in people with only mild insomnia, who would be just as likely to benefit from good sleep hygiene.

Often, the professional treatment of insomnia requires nothing more than various aspects of sleep hygiene. Sedentary insomniacs may be urged to take up daily regimens of vigorous exercise. Frequent nappers may be instructed to eat a light breakfast and lunch to reduce daytime drowsiness. A significant number of patients, however, need more than hygienic measures. Insomnia arising from psychiatric disorders may require extended investigation and treatment of the underlying problem. And some patients need special evaluation at a sleep clinic—especially those with symptoms of sleep apnea.

SLEEP APNEA—DEADLY SNORING

Sleep apnea is a potentially life-threatening syndrome accompanied by loud snores, violent snorts, and desperate gaspings for breath. Most commonly, it involves an obstruction of the upper airway during sleep; in other cases, the respiratory muscles temporarily stop working. Victims of the ailment may stop breathing anywhere from dozens to hundreds of times a night. Despite the disruptive episodes, sleep-apnea victims are usually unaware of their plight. Pronounced daytime drowsiness is usually the only telltale clue—although chronic insomnia is another possible symptom in some cases.

Severe sleep apnea can cause death from cardiac arrhythmias that may occur during an episode. Alcohol and sleep medications can prolong the apnea and may increase the risk of death as a result. The condition occurs most commonly in obese people, especially men. The frequency among women increases with age.

People who experience excessive daytime sleepiness without apparent cause should suspect sleep apnea, particularly if they are heavy snorers. (An estimated 2.5 million of the roughly 30 million American snorers experience sleep apnea.) Bedmates may be aware of the episodes that the victim sleeps through. If so, an immediate visit to a physician is in order. Patients with symptoms of sleep apnea will often be referred to a sleep-disorders center, where the diagnosis can be confirmed and the exact cause pinpointed.

Treatments for sleep apnea include medication, weight loss, and surgery. Many patients also obtain relief from a mechanical device, worn like a face mask, that forces air through the nose and prevents obstruction of the airway during sleep.

WHEN TO VISIT A SLEEP CLINIC

If good sleep hygiene and your physician's best efforts fail to relieve your insomnia, then it's time to consider a sleep clinic. During your initial evaluation, specialists in neurology, psychiatry, and pulmonary medicine may interview you, take your medical and psychiatric history, and review your symptoms and complaints. The findings will suggest whether you need any of several overnight tests. During sleep, the tests record various physical responses such as brain waves, breathing, and eye and muscle movements. The results help to identify the source of your insomnia and offer clues for appropriate therapy.

Sleep clinics are run by many large medical centers. An initial consultation and evaluation can cost anywhere from $50 to $300. Laboratory testing, such as an overnight sleep study, adds considerably more (some tests can cost nearly $1000). Most are covered by medical insurance, but insurance companies vary in their reimbursement policies. Be sure to check your coverage in advance.

DIET
and
NUTRITION

Diet and Your Heart

Like an endless courtroom drama, the role of diet in coronary heart disease has been hotly contested for nearly two generations. The indictment of the American diet as a possible malefactor was first drawn up in the years following World War II. Since then, a procession of scientists has taken the stand, presenting masses of data on the menus and bloodstreams of populations around the world.

Until 1984, the outcome of this scientific debate had been a succession of hung juries. Then the results of a long-awaited study were published. Called the Lipid Research Clinics Coronary Primary Prevention Trial (CPPT), the study showed that reducing abnormally high levels of cholesterol in the blood could reduce the incidence of heart attacks.

To the American Heart Association (AHA), the findings of the CPPT provided "smoking gun" evidence for dietary changes. The AHA has long advocated what is commonly known as the "prudent diet." It involves specific dietary measures to reduce the risk of heart disease, such as lowering the percentage of total dietary fat and choosing polyunsaturated fats over saturated fats. Saturated fats, which come primarily from foods of animal origin, tend to raise blood cholesterol levels. Polyunsaturated fats, which come mainly from vegetable sources, tend to lower blood cholesterol.

The link between coronary disease and blood cholesterol levels has been established by other studies of various population groups around the world. Groups with low blood cholesterol generally had lower rates of heart attack than those with high levels of blood cholesterol. At the same time, dietary experiments conducted with subjects in controlled settings suggest that there is a link between diet and blood cholesterol levels. In such studies, blood cholesterol levels can be influenced by the type of fat eaten and, to a lesser extent, by the amount of cholesterol consumed.

Logically, then, it appears that reducing the level of blood cholesterol—through diet, drugs, or other means—might reduce the risk of coronary heart disease. To physicians, this concept is known as the "lipid hypothesis." To people familiar with the AHA's dietary advice, it's the diet-heart theory.

Whatever the name, the ultimate goal is to prevent, retard, or even reverse the development of atherosclerosis—the buildup of fibrous, fatty deposits, called *plaques,* on the inner walls of major arteries. Atherosclerosis can reduce or cut off the blood flow in arteries serving major organs such as the heart or brain. When it affects the coronary arteries nourishing the heart, it can lead to heart attack and impaired heart function.

ELUSIVE PROOF

A theory requires proof before it can be accepted as fact. And, for many years, that proof remained elusive. More than a score of clinical trials failed to show convincingly that reducing blood cholesterol by diet or drugs reduced the incidence of a first heart attack. Yet a number of studies had strongly suggested that a change in diet could lower the incidence of second heart attacks.

Cholesterol, technically a sterol similar in structure to vitamin D and certain bile constituents, is found in all body cells and serves a number of important functions. It is a building block for cell membranes and steroid hormones, and it shares in other essential bodily processes. It's also an important component of arterial plaque, although its exact role in plaque formation is unclear.

Some of the clinical trials suggested that reducing blood cholesterol was beneficial. But, partly because of design weaknesses in many of the studies, the overall results were mixed and inconclusive.

Accordingly, even though several federal agencies and expert panels have advised cutting back on fat and cholesterol, many physicians tended to be skeptical. In a 1983 survey of 1600 physicians by the National Heart, Lung, and Blood Institute (NHLBI), which sponsored the CPPT study, 90 percent said that quitting smoking would have a "large impact" on the prevention or control of coronary disease and 80 percent said that reducing high blood pressure would—but only 39 percent said the same about reducing blood cholesterol levels. By the time a follow-up study was conducted in 1986, however, 64 percent of the physicians agreed with that statement about cholesterol.

The CPPT Study

Many public-health officials credit the CPPT results for changing minds about the importance of dietary measures to control cholesterol. Ironically, the study involved the test of a drug rather than diet. Nevertheless, it offers the strongest evidence to date for the value of blood-cholesterol reduction by any means. Even the CPPT's critics agree that the study was well designed and well executed. But there is disagreement over how the results should be interpreted.

The CPPT involved 3800 middle-aged men. All had blood cholesterol levels of at least 265 milligrams (per deciliter of blood)—enough to put them in the highest 5 percent of cholesterol levels among adult Americans. Although all were free of any sign of coronary disease on entry into the trial, they were considered to be at risk of heart attack because of their elevated cholesterol levels. (In the Framingham Heart Study, a long-running study of residents of Framingham, Massachusetts, men with an average blood cholesterol of 260 milligrams have experienced a heart attack rate three times as high as men with levels below 195. The average blood cholesterol among all Americans is 210 milligrams.)

The CPPT participants were randomly assigned to a treatment or a control group of 1900 men each. The treatment group took daily doses of a cholesterol-reducing drug, cholestyramine, while the controls received an indistinguishable placebo. *Both* groups followed a cholesterol-reducing diet for an average of 7.4 years. Over the course of the trial, the treatment group had fewer heart attacks than the control group (155 versus 187) and fewer deaths from heart attack (30 versus 38). Because of the large number of participants, the difference between the two groups was found to be statistically significant.

Taken in conjunction with other evidence, said the National Heart, Lung, and Blood Institute, the findings "support the view that cholesterol lowering by diet also would be beneficial." According to the NHLBI, the results could be "narrowly interpreted" to apply only to the use of a specific drug in middle-aged men with cholesterol levels above 265 milligrams. "The trial's implications, however, could and should be extended to other age groups and to women."

The NIH Panel's Verdict: Reduce Blood Cholesterol

Those recommendations drew little criticism—or even much attention—until late 1984, when the NHLBI joined in convening a panel of medical and public-health experts to address key questions about lowering blood cholesterol. Such meetings, called "consensus development conferences," are held periodically at the National Institutes of Health (NIH) to thrash out reasonable policies on controversial health issues. In this instance, the panel reached a unanimous verdict, coming out wholeheartedly for reducing blood cholesterol levels, *especially* by diet.

It has been established "beyond a reasonable doubt," said the NIH panel, that lowering elevated blood cholesterol levels will reduce the risk of heart attacks from coronary disease. "This has been demonstrated most conclusively in men with elevated blood cholesterol levels, but much evidence justifies the conclusion that similar protection will be afforded in women with elevated levels." The panel recommended that all individuals with blood cholesterol levels judged to be in high-risk or moderate-risk categories receive dietary treatment, and if necessary, drug treatment to reduce those levels. It defined the two categories in terms of blood cholesterol levels at specific ages (see chart, page 91).

The panel also concluded that blood cholesterol levels of most Americans are "undesirably high," largely because of high dietary intake of "calories, saturated fat, and cholesterol." It advised that all Americans except children under two follow a diet identical to the latest version of the American Heart Association's prudent diet. Children under two were excluded because of possible deleterious effects on normal growth and development.

The Recommended Diet

Specifically, the diet would pare fat intake to 30 percent of total calories consumed (from an average of about 40 percent now) and cut saturated fats to less than 10 percent of calories. Polyunsaturated fats would be limited to 10 percent of calories, and daily cholesterol intake would be held to 250 to 300 milligrams (roughly the amount in one egg). Total calories would also be reduced, if necessary, to correct obesity and maintain ideal body weight.

In practical terms, the diet means eating more fruit, vegetables, and grain products, and much less food from animal sources—especially fatty meats, dairy products, eggs, and rich baked goods. It also means favoring fish and poultry over beef, lamb, and pork, and limiting portions to roughly 4 to 6 ounces.

The panel based its conclusions on various types of evidence, including experimental animal data and population studies as well as clinical trials. One study sponsored by the NHLBI, for example, had shown that treatment with cholestyramine helped to slow the progression of arterial plaques in middle-aged male cardiac patients with elevated cholesterol levels. However, the "keystone in the arch," as the panel chairman put it, was the CPPT.

MIXED SUPPORT FOR UNIVERSAL CHANGE IN DIET

Despite the unanimity on the NIH panel, other medical experts view this "keystone" as a shaky support—especially for the panel's sweeping dietary advice to the entire public. For one thing, there's disagreement over whether beneficial effects achieved with a drug can be assumed for diet as well. Some contend that a cholesterol-lowering diet would be similar in action to the drug cholestyramine; others voice the opposite view.

The biggest bone of contention between the panel and its critics has been whether findings in high-risk, middle-aged men should be applied to the public at large. Virtually all clinical trials of cholesterol-lowering therapy have focused on middle-aged men. There's only limited clinical evidence available about the effects of reducing blood cholesterol in women or older people. And there's none at all for children or for people without elevated cholesterol levels. No one knows for sure whether reducing cholesterol levels in these groups is beneficial, harmful, or irrelevant.

Another study sponsored in part by the NHLBI was reported in 1987. Called the Cholesterol-Lowering Atherosclerosis Study (CLAS), it tested the effect of a similar cholesterol-lowering drug therapy on 162 middle-aged men who had previously undergone coronary bypass surgery. The control group received a placebo and followed the AHA diet; the treatment group received colestipol and niacin and followed an even more rigorous diet. Rather than counting heart attacks and deaths, the CLAS used angiograms (X rays of blood vessels) to evaluate the effect of treatment at the level of the arterial wall.

The results showed significant benefits from treatment. "Deterioration in overall coronary status was significantly less in drug-treated subjects than placebo-treated subjects." Actual improvement in coronary status was noted in 16 percent of the treatment group, as opposed to only 2 percent of the controls. The results indicated that actual regression of atherosclerosis is possible and demonstrated, for the first time, "a logical, mechanical explanation for benefits from blood cholesterol-lowering therapy."

"At this time," the researchers concluded, "we advocate measures to lower blood cholesterol levels in all postcoronary bypass patients." Despite the select population studied, they stated that their results "also support and extend" the cholesterol-lowering treatment goals developed in 1984 by the NIH consensus development conference.

Still, the questions remain: How much can diet do alone? And how would individuals other than the classic middle-aged male respond?

The Evidence from Epidemiology

The rationale for advising dietary changes in untested groups is based partly on epidemiology, the medical specialty that investigates the incidence and suspected causes of disease in various populations. Since World War II, studies of populations around the world have shown strong relationships between dietary fat, blood cholesterol, and cardiovascular disease.

Statistical associations can identify potentially related factors, but they can't prove a cause-and-effect relationship. Heart-disease rates have been associated positively or negatively with many factors, ranging from smoking and wine consumption to national income and the number of cars per 100 people. Scientists take some of these associations seriously and dismiss others. Even a highly plausible association requires confirming evidence from other research. With most groups other than middle-aged men, confirming data from clinical trials are either sparse or nonexistent.

Next to population studies, the most significant evidence implicating diet in heart disease comes from animal experiments. Diets high in cholesterol and fat have produced a form of atherosclerosis in various species, including such primates as rhesus monkeys. There's no consistency of effect from species to species, however, or even within species. Animals vary widely in their response to such diets. Rhesus monkeys are mainly vegetarians. Meat-eaters such as dogs and cats show the least sensitivity to fat and cholesterol, while rabbits seemingly develop plaques if they trip over an Easter egg.

CHOLESTEROL LEVELS AND RISK

Age	Moderate Risk	High Risk
2–19	170–185 mg.*	Above 185 mg.*
20–29	201–220	Above 220
30–39	221–240	Above 240
40 and over	240–260	Above 260

*Milligrams of cholesterol per deciliter of blood. Source: NIH consensus development conference.

The Role of Other Risk Factors

Meanwhile, a number of other considerations complicate the issue of dietary influence in coronary disease.

Whereas the risk of lung cancer is dramatically increased by cigarette smoking, and high blood pressure strongly affects the risk of stroke, the risk of heart attack is influenced by many different factors. Cigarette smoking, high blood pressure, and elevated blood cholesterol are three major ones. Other influences include age, male gender, diabetes, a family history of heart disease, a sedentary life-style, decreased high-density lipoprotein cholesterol (see page 92), and possibly behavioral and social factors.

Consequently, while diet tends to get most of the press coverage, it's not nearly as crucial as advertised. True, it can affect the blood cholesterol level—but that's only one of several important risk factors in coronary disease.

A substantial part of the data showing the effects of dietary cholesterol or fat on blood cholesterol levels comes from "metabolic ward" studies—controlled experiments conducted in hospitals or similar settings, using formula diets with precise quantities of cholesterol or fat. In contrast, the effects of dietary cholesterol and fat are not as clear-cut among people eating ordinary foods on free-choice diets. A mixed diet contains a variety of substances that have opposing effects on blood cholesterol. So the effect of a food may not depend solely on the amount of fat or cholesterol in it.

Furthermore, while fat-controlled diets have reduced blood cholesterol in clinical trials, such reduction requires serious dedication and sustained effort—not merely switching from butter to margarine or cutting out a single food such as eggs.

Good Cholesterol and Bad Cholesterol

Another confounding factor is the distribution of cholesterol in the blood. This involves HDL and LDL, sometimes popularly referred to as "good cholesterol" and "bad cholesterol."

Cholesterol circulates in the blood linked to large molecules called apoproteins, or carrier proteins. Low-density lipoprotein (LDL), a form of cholesterol-carrying protein in the apoprotein B family, seems to promote atherosclerosis by depositing cholesterol in the arterial wall. About two-thirds or more of total blood cholesterol is transported in LDL. High-density lipoprotein (HDL), part of the apoprotein A family, appears to protect against the disease process by removing cholesterol from the arterial wall. Increasing evidence now indicates that the relative distribution of cholesterol among those two types of lipoprotein is a better gauge of coronary risk than the total blood cholesterol level.

Some experts focus on the ratio of total cholesterol to HDL cholesterol. For example, a total cholesterol level of 240 milligrams might appear to represent a greater risk than a total level of 200 milligrams. Yet a person with a total level of 240 milligrams that is one-fourth HDL cholesterol (60 milligrams) would actually have a lower risk than a person with a 200-milligram level that is only one-fifth HDL (40 milligrams). So the person at 240 milligrams would have a ratio of 4 (240/60); the other person, a ratio of 5 (200/40). And the higher the ratio, the greater the risk.

The level of HDL cholesterol alone is also a strong indicator of coronary-disease risk. On average, the higher the level, the lower the risk.

Studies show that women, lean people, nonsmokers, people who consume two or more alcoholic beverages daily, and people who exercise regularly have relatively higher HDL levels than, respectively, men, obese people, smokers, nondrinkers, and sedentary people. A diet high in fat tends to increase both HDL and LDL, although not necessarily in the same proportions. Conversely, a low-fat diet tends to reduce both, again not necessarily in tandem.

A specific fraction of HDL cholesterol, called HDL_2, appears to be the part that is protective against heart attack. But the factors that raise or lower HDL_2 levels are not yet clear. Research suggests that an extended program of regular aerobic exercise raises HDL_2 and that moderate drinking does not. Quitting smoking also increased HDL_2 in one study.

More recently, the National Cholesterol Education Program, a group of experts convened to study policy, has decided to focus on LDL cholesterol. Individuals with LDL cholesterol less than 130 milligrams are considered to be at low risk. Those with levels between 130 and 160 are "borderline high," 160 to 190 "moderately high," and above 190 milligrams at "very high" risk. Currently, however, it is technically difficult to measure LDL cholesterol; determinations are arrived at by calculation. There is probably no need to determine LDL cholesterol when total cholesterol is less than 200 milligrams.

Further investigation is needed about these factors and others—especially the effects of diet.

WHAT IS THE BEST MENU?

Both critics and advocates of dietary measures seem to agree on one point: Various types of diet might lower blood cholesterol, but no one knows for sure which diet is best.

The AHA's prudent diet is low in fat and cholesterol and emphasizes foods with complex carbohydrates, such as vegetables and fruit. The diets of Greenland Eskimos and the Japanese are high in fish and fish oils, which lower cholesterol and have other effects on blood. Diets high in polyunsaturates, as in some vegetarian diets, are another alternative, as are those associated with Mediterranean countries, which tend to be high in monounsaturated fats such as olive oil.

Each of these diets has been linked with low rates of coronary disease in at least some populations. But there is little information about how they compare with one another in efficacy and safety—or how consistently Americans would adhere to them.

Meanwhile, scientific investigation is continuing to refine prevailing ideas on the presumed advantages or disadvantages of specific foods. For example, in fat-controlled diets, cod, flounder, and other low-fat fish have been recommended over oily, fatty fish such as salmon and mackerel. But there is increasing evidence that the fatty fish may have a beneficial effect on coronary disease (see Chapter 9).

Similarly, monounsaturated fats were long thought to be neutral in their effect on blood cholesterol. But recent research suggests that they can have a cholesterol-lowering effect similar to that of polyunsaturates—without lowering HDL levels as polyunsaturates do. This finding may give a boost to such products as olive oil at the expense of safflower oil and corn oil.

In addition to advising reductions in total and saturated fat, current AHA guidelines recommend limiting dietary cholesterol to 250 to 300 milligrams a day. In effect, that can mean only two or three eggs per week, since an egg contains roughly 250 milligrams of cholesterol. A public-health approach that discourages cholesterol consumption might well benefit people who are sensitive to cholesterol in their diet. But for other people, dietary cholesterol in itself has minimal, if any, adverse effects on blood cholesterol, even with moderate egg consumption.

The body, in fact, produces cholesterol on its own—about 800 to 1500 milligrams daily. Generally, when a person eats more cholesterol, the body responds by producing less. When a person eats less cholesterol, the body produces more. That natural response helps to regulate blood cholesterol levels. It doesn't work efficiently, though, in a significant number of people—and these are the ones who might benefit from limiting dietary cholesterol.

Eggs are relatively low in calories and high in important nutrients, making them especially suitable for diets to reduce obesity. Weight loss among people who are overweight is one of the most effective ways to reduce blood cholesterol. Paring excess weight also helps to lower high blood pressure and control diabetes—two other risk factors for coronary disease.

A PRUDENT APPROACH TO THE PRUDENT DIET

Despite various unanswered questions about the prudent diet, it deserves consideration by men with moderate or high levels of blood cholesterol as a possible risk-reducing measure. It avoids extremes and aims for a balanced variety of nutrients. It is unlikely to harm this population, and it may do some good.

A similar diet was used for some 1200 high-risk men in a five-year clinical trial in Oslo, Norway. That study reported a significant reduction in heart-attack rates, but the benefit from diet is difficult to assess because the trial included smoking reduction as well. There were no apparent ill effects from the diet.

For men with "low-risk" blood cholesterol levels, there's less to gain from the prudent diet, and there's no proof as yet that it will reduce their already low coronary risk. There's also little likelihood of harm for those who want to try the diet as a way of hedging their bets. However, a cholesterol-lowering diet is inadvisable for men with total blood cholesterol below 180 milligrams. In some epidemiological studies, cholesterol levels below that level are associated with a higher risk of mortality from causes other than coronary disease, particularly colon cancer.

For women, the possible value of the prudent diet is still unclear. There is little information about the effects of cholesterol-lowering therapy in women, and no clinical studies at all about the efficacy or safety of the diet for them. Women of any age have a lower risk of heart attack than their male counterparts. The difference is especially pronounced before menopause. Among white American adults under 45, for example, men have about 10 times the heart-attack rate of women.

Many women not only have less to gain from a fat-controlled diet, but in fact may incur more risk from it than men do. Meat and dairy foods, the targets for major cholesterol cutbacks, are important sources of iron and calcium, two nutrients that are already inadequate or marginal in many women's diets.

Despite such considerations, however, women with elevated blood cholesterol levels are at increased risk of coronary disease. Although there's no proof that the AHA diet will be beneficial, it's a reasonable precaution for women with levels in the high-risk or moderate-risk range, particularly after menopause.

CAUTIONS FOR CHILDREN AND THE ELDERLY

Perhaps the most controversial AHA recommendation is to extend the prudent diet to children two years of age and older. The NIH panel endorses that policy, but the American Academy of Pediatrics does not. Both groups agree on modifying diets for children with abnormally high cholesterol levels or inherited metabolic disorders. The disagreement centers on what healthy children should eat.

The main reason for starting a low-fat diet at age two is to foster that eating habit. "It is desirable to begin prevention in childhood because patterns of lifestyle are developed in childhood," the NIH panel said. Moreover, a specific diet may be easier to adhere to if all family members eat the same foods.

The American Academy of Pediatrics disagrees with that approach. Alvin M. Mauer, M.D., chairman of the Academy's committee on nutrition, spoke to CU in 1985. "There is no evidence that diet in childhood influences the development of atherosclerosis in adult men," he said. "Is it necessary to start the diet in childhood rather than in the early twenties?" The American Academy of Pediatrics has recently altered its view and recommends that children with elevated blood cholesterol levels be counseled on diet. What worried Mauer is that dietary restrictions may compromise growth and development, not only in young children, but also during the major growth spurt of adolescence. "Meat and eggs are good sources of iron and other nutrients needed for expanding blood volume and muscle growth," he said. "Dairy foods are a major source of calcium needed for bone development." Mauer also pointed out that the concept of family meals applies more to young children than to adolescents, most of whom eat only one meal a day at home.

Pediatricians who support adopting the AHA diet in children are confident that it's adequate for growth and development. But until enough experience is logged with high-risk children receiving dietary treatment, this assumption may be premature.

Caution is also warranted at the opposite end of the life span. The elderly often have special nutrition problems, including that of simply obtaining a balanced diet. Eggs, for example, are high in cholesterol, but they are also nutritious and cheap. Moreover, dental problems, chronic disorders, and economic or social constraints may partly dictate food choices. What older people may need least is another set of restrictions on what they should or shouldn't eat—particularly since the prudent diet hasn't been tested in this age group.

Meanwhile, people who want to try the AHA diet as a possible risk-reducing measure should bear in mind that it's not a self-sufficient program. Elimination of cigarette smoking, control of high blood pressure and diabetes, avoidance of a sedentary life-style, and reduction of obesity should all be part of a comprehensive program to reduce the risk of coronary disease.

Measurement of blood cholesterol, including its HDL and LDL fractions, should be one part of any overall evaluation of coronary risk. Since laboratory measurement may vary, at least two separate determinations should be made before accepting a value as accurate.

Seafood and Heart Disease

The nomadic hunters of the North American Arctic called themselves *Inuit,* which simply means "the people." Their more familiar name—Eskimos—comes from their ancient enemies, the Cree. It means "people who eat raw meat."

Raw or cooked, the traditional Eskimo diet—seal, whale, fish, caribou, and other Arctic wildlife—has become in the past few years the unlikely springboard for a new surge in dietary advice. Increasingly, medical and nutrition specialists are encouraging Americans to eat more fish in the hope of reducing the risk of heart attack. And, unlike earlier advice, which stressed "lean" fish for cholesterol watchers, the new consensus is that any fish—lean or fatty, finfish or shellfish—will do. In fact, it seems the fatter, the better.

Classic Eskimo fare would appear to be a cardiologist's nightmare. It's very high in animal fat and cholesterol and nearly devoid of vegetables, fruit, and grain. Yet heart disease is uncommon among Eskimos. Their blood cholesterol levels tend to be relatively low, with high concentrations of "good cholesterol" (high-density lipoprotein, or HDL, discussed in Chapter 8). One reason for this paradox is the type of fat Eskimos consume. Beef and pork, both staples of the traditional American diet, are relatively high in saturated fat, which tends to raise blood cholesterol. The fat of an Arctic seal or whale is much less saturated. It's more akin to fish oil, which is rich in monounsaturated and polyunsaturated fatty acids, which tend to lower blood cholesterol.

That much has been known since the early 1950s, when detailed analyses of the Eskimo diet began to appear in scientific journals. But when physicians advocated fish in cholesterol-reducing diets, their preference was for lean varieties, such as cod and flounder. So-called fatty fish like salmon were assigned the same pariah status as lard and egg yolk. Shellfish, considered high in cholesterol, were also frowned upon.

Today, research originating with studies of the Eskimos in the late 1970s has now cast an entirely new light on fish oils and their effects on body chemistry. Concurrent investigation has also brought shellfish back to the cholesterol-conscious consumer's menu.

FAT FISH AND THIN BLOOD

During the 1970s, Danish researchers observed that the Eskimos of northwest Greenland exhibited a mild bleeding disorder: They bruised easily and tended to experience nosebleeds. Subsequent investigation revealed that their platelets—blood cells involved in clotting—were less sticky than those of Europeans or Americans, and didn't clump together as readily. This finding suggested that the Eskimos' apparent resistance to coronary disease might be linked to the difference in their platelets. It may be that less-sticky platelets are less likely to form a clot, or "thrombus," that could cause a heart attack by blocking a coronary artery.

Whatever is affecting platelet function may also be serving to protect Eskimos from coronary disease. That hidden factor, it now appears, may be the Eskimos' high intake of certain fatty acids in their diet.

All fats, solid or liquid, are composed of various combinations of fatty acids. The types and amounts of acids present are what make one fat different from another. One group of polyunsaturated fatty acids—called the omega-6 group—is abundant in land plants. Another—the omega-3 group—is more plentiful in sea plants, especially in cold waters.

Omega-3 fatty acids typically remain liquid at extremely low temperatures. As it turns out, this is providential for both fish and sea mammals, particularly those that inhabit the Arctic. Omega-3 fatty acids are critical for maintaining the flexibility of the animals' cell membranes—which enables seals and fish to move about in their characteristic floppy way, rather than stiffly or not at all.

Fish are a good source of omega-3 fatty acids because they eat sea plants—or eat other fish that do. Generally, the colder the water and the oilier the fish, the greater the omega-3 content.

Like other fatty acids, the omega-3 variety enter the membranes of many body cells, including the platelets. The two omega-3 acids most common in fish oil are eicosapentaenoic acid and docosahexaenoic acid, or EPA and DHA. Research now indicates that sufficient intake of EPA and DHA can make platelets less "sticky"—and less likely to form clots. This effect on platelets is not confined to the Eskimo diet. Japanese fishermen who consume large amounts of fish daily also exhibit reduced platelet stickiness. Like the Eskimos, these fish-eaters experience a very low rate of coronary disease.

Part of the recent research has served to retire former misconceptions about fish. Fatty fish, for example, were supposed to raise blood cholesterol. They don't. Studies at the Oregon Health Sciences University showed that experimental diets high in fish oil and salmon (a fatty fish) actually lower the level of cholesterol in the blood somewhat. Such diets also dramatically reduce the blood level of triglycerides—fatty substances that are suspected of playing a role in coronary disease.

Moreover, the term *fatty* applied to fish is something of a misnomer. In the total universe of fat things, fish tend to be rather svelte. Overall, oily fish—salmon, mackerel, bluefish, lake trout, sardines, herring, and the like—have only about one-fifth to one-half the average fat content of lean beef.

Shellfish are very low in fat, often having less than the white meat of chicken. But they were long thought to be high in cholesterol and therefore inappropriate for people with elevated blood cholesterol. The first clue that this might not be so came in the late 1960s, when scientists at Oregon Health Sciences University tested the effects of shellfish in a dietary study. Participants who ate approximately a pound of shrimp, lobster, and crab daily for several weeks experienced little rise in blood cholesterol. When the diet shifted to mollusks—oysters, scallops, and clams—the participants actually showed a slight decrease in blood cholesterol.

The results were so unexpected that the researchers decided to shelve the study. When they finally published it in 1982, they explained that they had not submitted the data initially because they had not understood it. But recent insights had made some sense of the puzzling results.

Among those insights was a more accurate measure of the cholesterol in shellfish. Previous analytical techniques had identified marine substances similar to cholesterol as cholesterol itself. As a result, the cholesterol content of many shellfish had been greatly exaggerated.

More recent analyses by the U.S. Department of Agriculture have revised the numbers sharply downward, especially for mollusks. The formerly maligned sea scallop, for example, has not only about half the fat of white-meat chicken, but less cholesterol as well. Even some popular crustaceans score reassuring marks. The cholesterol level of crab and lobster is roughly comparable to the dark meat of chicken and is much lower in fat. Shrimp tends to be higher in cholesterol than other shellfish and most meat, but only moderately so.

CONFIRMATION FROM RECENT FINDINGS

The succession of favorable reports reached a peak in 1985 when the *New England Journal of Medicine* published three studies supporting the possible benefits of seafood. Prominently featured was a report from the Netherlands concluding that fish consumption might lower the risk of fatal heart attack.

Some 850 men in the town of Zutphen had been followed for 20 years to assess various risk factors in heart disease. A major finding was that fish consumption was associated with a reduced rate of fatal coronaries. Men who ate roughly 7 to 11 ounces of fish weekly had less than half the coronary death rate of men who ate no fish at all. Men who consumed more than 11 ounces of fish a week—about a pound, on average—experienced virtually the same reduction in risk as those who ate 7 to 11 ounces. There was no extra advantage to the higher level of intake.

Even when other common risk factors such as hypertension, smoking, and elevated blood cholesterol were taken into account, the favorable association with fish intake persisted. The Dutch researchers concluded that "as little as one or two fish dishes per week may be of preventive value in relation to coronary heart disease."

In its implications for U.S. public health, the Dutch study was more provocative than the findings among Eskimos or Japanese fishermen. The Japanese consumed more than half a pound of fish daily. Eskimos may have eaten the equivalent of nearly a pound a day. But the Dutch ate fish in amounts that Americans might well get used to eating. One or two fish meals a week is well within range of a health-conscious public. Even though the Dutch findings only suggest—rather than prove—that fish is good for the heart, there's still ample room for more fish as part of a well-balanced American diet.

FISH OIL CAPSULES

Besides urging more patronage at the fish counter, public-health officials generally agree on another issue. They want people to eat fish rather than swallow fish-oil capsules.

Wide press coverage of the research on fish oil helped create a popular item in the food-supplement market. Capsules of fish oil containing marine fatty acids—especially EPA and DHA—were suddenly peddled to people hoping to gain an edge on heart disease, arthritis, or other assorted maladies.

Fish oil is admittedly more than just snake oil with gills. Large doses of marine fatty acids given both as salmon oil and as fish-oil capsules have shown promise for lowering excessive levels of triglycerides in the blood. There's also evidence that such doses may have an anti-inflammatory effect by inhibiting certain biochemical processes in white blood cells. But research is preliminary and contradictory, and little is known about actual clinical benefits.

Also unknown is the extent of adverse effects—which may include diarrhea and delayed blood clotting. (People on aspirin therapy or taking anticoagulants should avoid fish-oil capsules.) One certain side effect is cost: The manufacturers' "recommended daily dose" of fish-oil supplements can run you anywhere from $10 to $40 or more per month—and even that would not be enough to approach the level of fatty acids found to be beneficial in clinical studies.

There's no proof as yet that taking a daily fish-oil capsule or two will do anything more than grease your intestines. Pending further clinical trials, most researchers advise eating fish instead.

CAUTIONS

Meanwhile, the possible dark side to a high-fish diet needs to be explored. Inhibited platelet function isn't necessarily a sign of bristling health.

Changing the body's fatty-acid makeup may have effects, good and bad, that are still uncharted. For example, there's some evidence that Eskimos and Japanese fishermen experience higher death rates from brain hemorrhage than Europeans or Americans do. Some scientists suggest that the difference could be related to inhibition of platelet function. Some people are allergic to fish, becoming ill from eating even a small amount.

For most people, however, there isn't much to worry about in a couple of fish meals a week.

Most problems arise when fish come from contaminated waters. If you're fond of raw shellfish, for example, it's difficult to avoid some risk of hepatitis or food poisoning. If shellfish come from an area where outbreaks have been traced to them, avoid eating any raw. Always steam clams for at least four to six minutes, not just until the shell opens.

Eating raw fish, such as preparations of Japanese sushi or sashimi, also involves a risk, mainly from an intestinal parasite known as the fish tapeworm. Although ocean fish usually present no problem, lake fish and Alaskan salmon are sometimes infected. Accordingly, if you prepare raw fish yourself, stick to ocean varieties. In restaurants, inquire about the source of fish before ordering.

Commercially sold fish come under federal regulations that strictly limit them to extremely low levels of mercury, pesticide residues, or other contaminants. Those regulations don't apply to sport fish, however. If you eat sport fish frequently, try to avoid those from lakes or streams known to have pollution problems.

Current limits on the amount of mercury in commercial fish are designed to protect fetuses, which are most vulnerable to mercury toxicity. Even so, it's possible for a pregnant woman to exceed the permissible level for mercury intake—and transmit the contaminant to the fetus—if she eats a lot of fish, particularly large predators such as swordfish, tuna, red snapper, freshwater trout, and northern pike.

Salt and Your Health

The suspected role of salt in promoting high blood pressure is well seasoned with controversy. Is salt—or the sodium it contains—really such a villain? How does it affect your body and your health? And with high levels of sodium all around you, how can you avoid it? Should you bother?

SALT AND HIGH BLOOD PRESSURE

Salt, or sodium chloride, is a health issue because of its sodium content. Sodium plays a major role in the regulation of body fluids and is commonly assumed to have an influence on blood pressure. The main source of sodium in the American diet, salt is about 40 percent sodium. Other typical sources include various food additives, such as monosodium glutamate (MSG), sodium phosphate, and sodium nitrite. Sodium is also a natural component of many foods, as well as an ingredient in many processed foods and some medicines.

Everyone needs some sodium in the diet to replace routine losses. About 200 milligrams a day is considered an essential amount for survival; individual requirements vary with physical activity, climate, and other factors. The Food and Nutrition Board of the National Academy of Sciences/National Research Council estimates that an "adequate and safe" intake of sodium for healthy adults is 1100 to 3300 milligrams a day, the equivalent of approximately ½ to 1½ teaspoons of salt. Americans generally consume at least twice that amount. Estimated intakes of individuals range from 2300 to 6900 milligrams of sodium daily, according to the Food and Nutrition Board.

Most people appear to suffer no ill effects from a high salt intake. But a significant minority—the roughly 20 percent of American adults who develop high blood pressure—can be adversely affected by excessive amounts of sodium in their diets. Their sodium intake influences their blood-pressure levels, and some researchers believe it may contribute to the development of the condition.

High blood pressure, or hypertension, is a persistent elevation of blood pressure above normal levels. (The term *tension* here refers to pressure, not to nervous tension; both tense and seemingly relaxed people can be susceptible to hypertension.) If the disease is not detected and treated, it can eventually lead to stroke, heart attack, or kidney failure. For purposes of diagnosis and treatment, hypertension is commonly defined as mild, moderate, or severe.

Until recently, advice to cut back on sodium was directed primarily to people with hypertension or to those considered at risk of developing it. The latest recommendations, however—and the advertising campaigns they prompted—are aimed at the American public in general. In 1980, dietary guidelines issued jointly by the U.S. Department of Agriculture and Department of Health and Human Services began to advocate that all Americans "moderate" their sodium intake. Similar advice is offered by several health or science groups, such as the American Heart Association and the National Heart, Lung, and Blood Institute. The recommended sodium intake varies or is sometimes left unstated, but all those groups agree the intake should go down.

Despite such official blessings, the call for a sodium cutback for the public at large has not drawn universal applause. Among experts on hypertension, reaction to the federal guidelines ranges from enthusiastic support to heated criticism. While some view the advice as reasonable and practical, others argue that it's unwarranted and lacks adequate scientific justification.

At the crux of the debate is a question common to many public-health policies: Is it reasonable to prescribe something for an entire population to protect a vulnerable minority—in this case, the people susceptible to hypertension? The issue in this instance arouses further controversy because there is no proof that excess sodium actually *causes* hypertension or that lowering sodium intake will prevent the disease. By contrast, a public-health measure like childhood vaccination is widely accepted because it's known to be effective in preventing specific illnesses.

Long-term studies may resolve the sodium issue, but not in the near future. Accordingly, many people will have to decide whether cutting back on sodium makes good sense for them. In making an individual decision, it's important to understand what hypertension is, what role sodium might play, and whether you are in one of the "risk groups" that experience a higher incidence of the disease.

ANATOMY OF HYPERTENSION AND THE SUSPECTED ROLE OF SODIUM

The body regulates blood pressure through a complex system. The system works by means of nerve signals, hormones, and other influences to widen or narrow the arterioles—small, muscular blood vessels that carry oxygen and nutrients from the arteries to the tissues. If a part of the body needs a lot of nourishment at a particular time (the stomach during digestion, for example), nearby arterioles expand to allow increased blood flow. Arterioles in other parts of the body constrict to maintain normal blood pressure.

In some people, the regulatory system goes awry. Arterioles all over the body constrict at the same time and stay constricted. Pressure in the larger arteries goes up and stays up. The result is an abnormal, sustained rise in blood pressure.

In about 10 percent of hypertensive patients, the faulty regulatory effect is traceable to kidney disease, to localized narrowing of the arteries leading to the kidneys, or to a tumor or overactivity of the adrenal glands. Some of those problems may be corrected by surgery or by specific medications, after which blood pressure usually returns to normal.

In most cases of hypertension, however, the cause of the regulatory breakdown is obscure. When the cause is unknown, the condition is called *essential hypertension.*

Some researchers believe that the unknown cause is high salt consumption. As evidence, they point to studies of salt intake in animals and humans.

In the early 1960s, Lewis K. Dahl of Brookhaven National Laboratory discovered that a high salt intake caused elevated blood pressure in about three-quarters of the laboratory rats he fed salted feed. The rest weren't affected. Through breeding, Dahl then produced two distinct strains of rats: a sensitive strain that developed severe high blood pressure from salted feed, and a resistant strain that ate the same amount of salt but maintained normal pressures. He concluded that the adverse response to salt was inherited. Dahl also made another observation: The blood pressures of the genetically susceptible rats remained normal on a diet very low in salt.

Many hypertension authorities believe that people react to salt in much the same way as Dahl's rats. Some are resistant to hypertension and never develop the disease even though they eat large amounts of salt all their lives. Others appear to inherit a susceptibility to high blood pressure, and a high-salt diet seems to promote the disease. If this theory is correct, susceptible people may be able to avoid hypertension by using salt sparingly throughout life.

For obvious reasons, clinical studies comparable to those performed on rats have never been done with people. So, direct evidence as to whether a high-salt intake can cause hypertension in humans (or whether a low-salt diet can prevent it) doesn't exist.

Some indirect evidence is available, however. It comes mainly from studies of different populations that eat varying amounts of salt.

Some isolated tribes, such as the Kung Bushmen of the Kalahari Desert and the Yanomamo Indians of Brazil, consume diets extremely low in salt, generally less than 500 milligrams a day. Studies of such tribes have found that the people experience virtually no hypertension and that their blood pressures do not rise with age, as do those of people in industrialized societies. In contrast, farmers in northern Japan, who preserve food with salt, consume as much as 30 *grams* of salt daily (about six teaspoons). Approximately 40 percent of them have high blood pressure, and the most common cause of death is stroke.

Similar studies have been carried out on more than 20 cultures, ranging from Greenland Eskimos to natives of the Solomon Islands in the South Pacific. Taken together, the studies show that hypertension is rare in populations that use very little salt. Conversely, in societies where a lot of salt is consumed, a significant minority of the people develop the disease.

Such studies *suggest*—but don't prove—that salt intake is related to essential hypertension in humans. Skeptics point out that the cultures that do not experience hypertension are all primitive or nonindustrial people whose salt intake is hardly the only thing that sets them apart from Americans. They are much leaner and more physically active than Americans, their diets differ in other ways, and they are free from various stresses of modern industrial life. Perhaps these factors, and not just a low-salt intake, would help to explain the lack of high blood pressure in such societies.

Meanwhile, the exact way that sodium influences blood pressure is still not firmly established. One view is that it affects blood-pressure levels through its ability to promote water retention and expand the body's fluid volume. This in turn produces increased pressure within the arteries. Another theory, which may or may not involve sodium, is that a generalized decrease in the diameter of the smaller blood vessels causes a resistance to blood flow that affects blood pressure.

Whether or not those theories are correct, virtually all authorities agree that low-sodium diets can reduce blood pressure in many patients with mild hypertension. What has not yet been established, however, is that a moderate cutback in sodium intake can *prevent* hypertension in susceptible people. For the majority of Americans, moreover, there's currently no evidence that the level of their salt intake affects their blood pressure at all.

In a study published in 1983, for example, researchers at Yale University School of Medicine examined the effect of salt intake on blood pressure among 3566 Connecticut residents who had never been diagnosed as hypertensive. All of the subjects were interviewed about their dietary salt intake and had their blood pressure recorded. After developing an approximate "index" of salt intake, the scientists compared the mean blood pressure of those in the top 10 percent of the salt-consumption index with the mean of those in the bottom 10 percent. The difference in average blood pressure between the heaviest and the lightest salt users was insignificant.

"These findings indicate that it is unlikely [that] dietary salt intake has a clinically significant effect on blood pressure in the majority of individuals in a large defined population," the researchers reported in the *Journal of the American Medical Association*. They also noted, however, that their findings would not rule out the possibility of a clinically significant effect for a minority of "salt-sensitive individuals."

RISK FACTORS FOR DEVELOPING HYPERTENSION

Despite evidence that as many as four out of five Americans probably needn't worry about their salt intake, a practical problem remains.

Although many people will never develop hypertension even if they eat relatively large amounts of salt all their lives, there's no way to tell in advance who they are. Nor is there any reliable means of predicting which individuals will be susceptible to hypertension. There are, however, certain risk factors that suggest which people are more likely than others to become hypertensive.

- A **family history** of hypertension is one warning signal. If either of your parents or a brother or sister has (or had) hypertension, you're about twice as likely to develop it as someone without such a history.
- **Race** is another factor. Black people are twice as likely as whites to develop hypertension. In blacks, the disease develops earlier in life, is often more severe, and is more likely to be fatal at a younger age than in whites. The hypertension rate for blacks age 25 to 34, for example, is about 19 percent, compared to about 8 percent for whites. And death rates from hypertension and hypertensive heart disease before age 50 are at least six times higher among blacks.
- **Obesity** can also influence blood pressure. About 30 percent of adult Americans are overweight. Studies show a higher prevalence of hypertension in overweight people than in lean people. Among overweight people who develop hypertension, weight loss is frequently one of the most effective ways to reduce blood pressure, often to normal levels. So counting calories may be just as important for an overweight person as watching salt intake.
- **Age** is another factor, for whites as well as blacks. In Western societies, blood pressure rises with age, and nearly half of all Americans who live to age 74 develop hypertension. Consequently, moderating salt intake may be a worthwhile precaution for older people.

LOW-SALT DIETS AND DRUG THERAPY

Physicians have known about the effect of low-salt diets since the 1940s, when drastic reductions of sodium intake were first used to treat severe cases of high blood pressure. But few patients could tolerate the monotonous fare, which had to be restricted to a few selections, such as rice, fruit, and sugar.

Such narrowly limited diets were largely abandoned in 1957, when thiazide diuretics were introduced for treating hypertension. Those drugs produced the same overall effect as sodium-restricted diets. By ridding the body of excess salt and water, they reduced the body's fluid volume and lowered blood pressure. Other drugs have since been developed to combat hypertension. Some reduced blood pressure by directly relaxing certain blood vessels and decreasing resistance to blood flow. Others blocked nerve impulses that indirectly raise blood pressure. Although hypertensive patients were still encouraged to "go easy on the salt," dietary treatment was largely replaced by the new drugs.

More recently, the low-sodium diet has attracted renewed interest, for a variety of reasons. Antihypertensive drugs can cause unpleasant side effects, leading some patients to stop the medication. Also, patients must take the drugs for the rest of their lives, and possible long-term side effects are an added concern.

Prescribing drugs to treat mild or "borderline" hypertension is still controversial. There's little doubt that even mild hypertension increases a person's risk of developing serious complications. Yet a number of hypertension specialists question whether the "costs" of drug treatment for mild hypertension—side effects, medical expense, and possible long-term hazards—are worth the presumed benefits. Evidence that drug treatment of mild hypertension reduces morbidity and mortality is not as convincing as that for treatment of moderate and severe hypertension.

Earlier use of drastic low-sodium diets was usually limited to people with severe hypertension. In recent years, though, researchers have tried less-restricted regimens on patients with mild or moderate hypertension. A number of patients have shown improvement with just a moderate decrease in their sodium intake. Some achieved normal blood pressure and no longer needed drugs. Others still had to take medication but could get by on lower doses, with fewer side effects.

The knowledge that patients often stray from low-sodium diets still leads many physicians to rely on drugs when treating hypertension. And prescribing drugs is easier than trying to persuade patients to change long-established eating habits. But recent success with moderate sodium restriction is convincing an increasing number of physicians that such restriction, along with several other nondrug measures, should be the initial treatment for mild hypertension.

And there is a growing trend to treat mild hypertension without drugs. Patients are being encouraged to make changes in life-style that may help to reduce blood pressure, such as losing weight if they're overweight, moderating alcohol intake, and getting regular exercise. An obvious advantage of this approach is that the recommended measures offer health benefits beyond their potential benefit in treating hypertension.

But long-standing habits are not easily changed, and a lifelong fondness for salt is no exception—expecially when there's so much of the stuff around. To effectively cut down on sodium in your diet, you have to know where to look.

REDUCING SODIUM IN YOUR DIET

Most people don't realize how pervasive sodium is in the American diet until they try to cut down.

Nature provides a more than adequate supply in foods of animal origin, in vegetables, and even in some water supplies. You can exceed the body's minimum daily requirement of about 200 milligrams without even trying. For instance, three ounces of lean cooked beef contains about 50 milligrams; half a cooked chicken breast, about 70 milligrams. One cup of milk contains about 120 milligrams of sodium, and an egg, about 60 milligrams. Raw celery, carrots, artichokes, and leafy greens such as chard, kale, and spinach range from 25 to 50 milligrams per half-cup.

The amount of sodium in a cup of drinking water generally ranges from less than 1 milligram to about 20 milligrams. The local water department can tell you the sodium content in your area's water supply. Water softeners add sodium to drinking water by replacing "hard" minerals with softer ones such as sodium. The harder the water, the more sodium your softener is adding. The amount of sodium added generally ranges up to about 25 milligrams per cup.

Overall, naturally occurring sodium accounts for only about one-third of the sodium in American diets. The rest comes from the salt people sprinkle on foods and the additives manufacturers include in processed foods.

Salt is known to be an acquired taste, and many families routinely add it in the cooking or at the table, perhaps as much out of habit as out of taste. Short of throwing away the salt shaker, how does someone who wants to cut down on sodium break the salt habit?

The first step is to reacquaint the taste buds with unsalted foods. Omit the salt used in cooking—you'll miss that the least. Instead, try using more flavorings, such as onion, and doubling the quantity of herbs you normally use. Once you are at the table, practice tasting the food before you reach for the salt.

Storing the salt shaker away from the table in an inconvenient location can also inhibit use. You might also try deceiving your salt cravings by using a shaker that has smaller or fewer holes.

It is not hard to get into the habit of using spices and herbs creatively, and there are numerous low-sodium cookbooks now that give guidelines for cooks. For example, with fish you can use a combination of such delicate herbs and spices as white pepper, lemon peel, celery seed, and poultry seasoning. With meat, you need a combination that's more hearty and robust: try black pepper, red bell peppers, celery seed, dry mustard, onion powder, garlic powder, thyme, oregano, and poultry seasoning. Avoid seasonings that come in salt form, though, such as garlic salt and onion salt; they are very high in sodium. Green vegetables such as snap beans, broccoli, and peas go well with basil, marjoram, tarragon, thyme, savory, mustard seed, rosemary, dill, or oregano. There are also premixed seasonings that you might try. But read the labels to make certain there is no sodium content.

Using a salt substitute may be another way to reduce sodium. These products generally use potassium chloride alone or with other seasonings to try to replace the taste of sodium chloride. But the unhappy fact is that potassium chloride doesn't taste much like salt. And many of the very people who must limit their sodium intake may also need to control potassium intake. If the potassium in their blood increases to harmful levels, serious disruption of normal heart function may result. Most salt substitutes now carry a warning on their labels to use only on advice of a physician. The average healthy adult interested in reducing sodium intake can safely use these products; normally functioning kidneys are capable of excreting excess potassium.

SODIUM AT THE SUPERMARKET

Anyone would recognize some processed foods as salty: olives, anchovies, dill pickles, sauerkraut, soy sauce, bacon, hot dogs, snack foods. Other high-sodium foods are not so obviously salty: tomato juice, cottage cheese, instant pudding, instant hot cereals.

Families who eat a lot of processed and convenience foods—and fast foods, for that matter—are consuming far more sodium than they need. One way for them to cut down might be to try some of the new lower-sodium foods now available in the supermarkets. These products are alternatives to processed foods that are traditionally high in sodium, such as potato chips, soups, peanut butter, and tomato sauce.

Sodium salts are an inexpensive way for manufacturers to enhance the flavor of foods that have lost natural flavor in processing; they are also used to preserve food. In processed meats, sodium salt may often be used to increase tenderness by inhibiting the hardening of muscle fibers in cooking and/or to increase water retention. In canned vegetables and fruits, salt may be used to preserve color or as a part of the processing. For instance, some vegetables are sorted in brine; the overripe ones sink and the less ripe ones float. Most canned whole tomatoes and some canned or frozen fruits are bathed in a caustic solution of sodium hydroxide to remove their peel. In baked goods, salt controls yeast fermentation rates and has a stiffening effect on dough, resulting in a firmer product. Other sodium salts in the form of baking soda and baking powder provide a gas in the dough that helps leaven baked goods.

Cheese contains a lot of sodium because salt plays such an important role in its processing. Sodium chloride retards the growth of undesirable organisms, helps coagulate the milk mix to form curds and whey, and also acts to develop flavor.

Manufacturers are reducing sodium in different ways, depending on the food. Some processed foods use sodium compounds as preservatives; manufacturers are now experimenting with other methods of preservation that may sometimes require you to refrigerate the product after opening. In foods that "need" salt to enhance what's left of natural flavors after processing, manufacturers are trying salt substitutes such as potassium chloride, various flavoring and seasoning ingredients, and sometimes complete reformulation of the recipe itself. Some foods—peanut butter, for instance—survive processing with most of their flavor intact, but have always been salted anyway. Now manufacturers are simply cutting out the salt.

How do you know the salt status of the foods you buy? Labels usually don't tell you how much salt has been added. In fact, sodium labeling, which is under the jurisdiction of the U.S. Food and Drug Administration (FDA), was until recently entirely voluntary unless the manufacturer made a sodium claim on the label. Now sodium content per serving must appear on all nutrition labels. (Remember, though, that "serving size" is determined by the manufacturer.)

The FDA has also adopted rules for the wording of sodium claims. According to these rules, "sodium free" means 5 milligrams or less of sodium per serving; "low sodium," 35 or less; "moderately low sodium," 140 or less. "Reduced sodium" indicates that the product has been reduced in sodium by 75 percent or more.

The medicine you take may also be a surprisingly high source of sodium—especially some over-the-counter drugs that are taken frequently over extended periods. Those include certain pain relievers, antacids, cough medicines, laxatives, and sedatives. For example, *Alka-Seltzer* with aspirin contains over 1000 milligrams of sodium per dose; *Rolaids* contains 106 milligrams per two-tablet dose. Some OTC drugs list sodium content on their labels; some are offered in versions with less sodium. For other drugs, your pharmacist or physician should be able to look up the sodium content for you.

11

Fiber and Colon Cancer

John Harvey Kellogg developed cornflakes to provide more "roughage" for the American diet. For years, cereals and other high-fiber foods have been promoted as healthful. And from time to time, the public has gone through waves of enthusiasm for increasing fiber in the diet.

In recent years, advertising for Kellogg's *All-Bran* has stoked the fiber furor with a vengeance. Kellogg's TV commercials have said explicitly that a high-fiber diet (and by implication, a diet featuring bran cereals) "may help to prevent certain kinds of cancer." The ads are correct—as far as they go. They would be more correct if the actor who delivers that line put a heavy stress on the word *may*.

Dietary fiber, or roughage, is the indigestible part of plant foods—fruits, vegetables, grains, and legumes. It adds bulk to the feces and may help to prevent constipation, hemorrhoids, and diverticulitis (a common, and occasionally serious, intestinal disorder). But those effects aren't what's making fiber famous. Rather, it's fiber's reported potential for reducing the risk of cancer of the colon.

Among all cancers, colon cancer is second only to lung cancer in its toll of American lives. Every year, the disease kills about 60,000 people. Every year, physicians diagnose some 90,000 new cases. Only about half of those diagnosed survive five or more years after diagnosis. So there's good reason indeed to pay attention to dietary measures that might reduce the risk of the disease.

In 1984, the U.S. Department of Health and Human Services said that if Americans ate less fat and more fiber, cases of colon cancer in the United States could fall by 30 percent, saving some 20,000 lives each year. The Canadian government, the U.S. Department of Agriculture, and the National Cancer Institute, among others, have also suggested that people should eat more fiber.

The official endorsements of fiber were quickly seized upon by product marketers. Store shelves are now stacked high with high-fiber breads, breakfast cereals, and packages of wheat, corn, and oat bran. The Kellogg's *All-Bran* campaign even boasts an implicit endorsement by the National Cancer Institute.

THE ANATOMY OF FIBER

Fiber comes from plants—in different amounts from different parts of different plants. A grain of wheat, for instance, contains about 12 percent fiber overall. But the grain's endosperm, the part millers grind to make white flour, is less than 4 percent fiber. The wheat grain's germ is about 13 percent fiber. And the bran that covers the outside of the wheat grain is more than 40 percent fiber. Whole-grain breads and bran cereals thus provide a great deal more dietary fiber than does white bread.

Further, dietary fiber consists of a number of different substances, which appear to affect the body in different ways. These substances can be divided into two types, soluble and insoluble. Soluble fiber dissolves in hot water; insoluble fiber does not. Some plant foods contain mostly soluble fiber, others mainly insoluble fiber. But virtually every food is a mixture; almost no foods provide a "pure form" of one type or the other.

Soluble fiber (pectin, gums, and some other substances) appears to have several beneficial effects. It adds bulk and thickness to the contents of the stomach and may slow emptying of the stomach, thus prolonging the sense of fullness and possibly helping dieters control their appetites. Studies have shown that soluble fiber lowers blood cholesterol levels somewhat. It also slows the absorption of sugars from the small intestine, which may be of benefit to diabetics.

Soluble fiber is readily available from a wide variety of grains, fruits, and vegetables. Good sources are prunes, pears, oranges, apples, dry beans, cauliflower, zucchini, sweet potatoes, and oat and corn bran.

However, there is little credible evidence that soluble fiber helps to prevent colon cancer. The evidence that exists points to insoluble fiber for possible protection.

Insoluble fiber includes cellulose, lignin, and hemicellulose (the last is also available as soluble fiber). The best sources of insoluble fiber are whole-grain cereals, especially wheat-bran cereals, and whole-grain breads.

Insoluble fiber adds bulk to the contents of the intestine, rather than the stomach. That speeds the passage—the "transit time"—of a meal's remnants through the small and large intestines. (That's why insoluble fiber helps prevent constipation.) The speedier passage through the colon may decrease the time that cells in the colon's lining are exposed to toxins—including carcinogens—that could be present, thus reducing the chances of colon cancer. Researchers have also proposed several other theories for the presumed protective effect of insoluble fiber. For example:

- Insoluble fiber may inactivate certain carcinogens or interfere with their effect.
- Insoluble fiber may lessen the production of bacterial enzymes that can convert bile acids into carcinogens.
- Insoluble fiber stimulates the secretion of mucus in the colon. Mucus coats the colon wall and may provide a barrier that keeps toxic substances, including carcinogens, from reaching the colon's cells.

THE EVIDENCE ON COLON CANCER

When CU wrote in 1981 about reports that a high-fiber diet may help to prevent colon cancer, we regarded it as a theory still far from proven. Unproven it remains. But in the years since then, evidence has continued to accumulate suggesting that appropriate amounts of fiber may have such a protective effect. Here's a look at what the evidence to date shows, and why it falls short of being conclusive.

Most of the evidence for the anticancer effect of fiber comes from epidemiological studies—that is, studies of diseases as they appear in populations of people. The first hint that fiber could protect against cancer came to public attention in 1974, when Denis P. Burkitt, a British physician, and his colleagues reported that rural Africans, who suffer much less colon cancer than Americans, typically consume much more fiber (50 to 150 grams per day) than do Americans (10 to 20 grams per day).

In another study, researchers found that Danes in Copenhagen, who consumed an average of 17 grams of fiber per day, suffered from three times as much colon cancer as the Finns of Kuopio, who consumed an average of 31 grams per day. Similar correlations have been shown in studies in Great Britain, Connecticut, and elsewhere, but not consistently.

In general, the key difference between the populations under study appeared to be in their consumption of insoluble fiber found in whole-grain cereals and whole-grain baked goods.

Also, people on vegetarian or semivegetarian diets—which often contain high levels of both soluble and insoluble fiber—have a low incidence of colon cancer.

Epidemiologists have found additional evidence for the anticancer effect of dietary fiber using the "case control" method. In this approach, researchers compare what colon-cancer patients say about their past diet with reports from noncancer subjects of similar age and background. Colon-cancer patients report having eaten significantly less fiber than do people without the disease.

Further evidence comes from animal research. Investigators have given rats various chemical carcinogens in their food or by injection while varying the animals intake of dietary fiber. In most of these studies, rats on high-fiber diets suffered fewer cancers than those on low-fiber diets. However, the results in rats have not been consistent; some studies found that the fiber had no effect, or even that it increased the cancer rate.

None of the evidence can be regarded as conclusive. The epidemiological evidence, for example, is subject to many possible interpretations. When comparing two population groups, such as Africans and Americans, there are always many differences between the groups, not only in diet but in several other aspects of life. So it's difficult to be certain that fiber consumption is the key variable. And people who eat more fiber tend to eat less of other things, particularly fat. High-fat and high-calorie diets have been shown by many researchers to increase the risk of several kinds of cancer, including colon cancer.

There is another difficulty in interpreting the epidemiological data. What appears to be a general effect of ingested fiber may turn out to be the effect of other components in certain foods. The cruciferous vegetables, for instance—broccoli, cabbage, kale, and brussels sprouts—have been shown in some studies to have a possible protective effect against colon cancer.

Case-control studies have problems, too. It is difficult for researchers to control for all possible variables that might have caused some patients to develop colon cancer while others remained free of the disease. In addition, people may not remember accurately what types of foods they ate years ago. (Then again, there is no reason to think that colon-cancer patients should differ from other people in their recall abilities.)

The animal experiments with rats are again suggestive rather than conclusive. As noted earlier, results have been mixed. And one can't always extrapolate reliably from the physiological reaction of one species to that of another. Moreover, even in the positive studies, not all kinds of fiber had the same protective effect, and the rats did not respond in the same way with all carcinogens.

Conflicting patterns in some earlier studies heighten the uncertainty. A few studies have reported that eating more fiber can be associated with a *greater* risk of colon cancer, in both rats and humans. One such report came from Australia in 1986. The researchers applied the case-control technique to 419 colon-cancer patients and 732 control subjects. They found that the colon-cancer patients had consumed slightly more cereal fiber than the controls had. The researchers narrowed down the increased cancer risk to older women, but their study may have broader implications.

Based on the Australian study and other research, some physicians believe that cancer might result from either too little or too much fiber. Many also stress the desirability of consuming fiber from a variety of sources, rather than relying on a single source.

Several of the studies on fiber are hard to interpret. Some studies—especially the older ones—fail to distinguish between soluble and insoluble fiber; there is preliminary evidence that some soluble fiber may actually increase cancer incidence. That evidence comes exclusively from rat studies involving relatively small numbers of test animals.

The issue warrants continued investigation, but does not justify changing your diet based on the risk—if any—that soluble fiber may present. At this time, CU's consultants recommend that total fiber consumption should include both soluble and insoluble fiber. But be sure that insoluble fiber constitutes a fair part of the mix.

As research on fiber intensifies, more uncertainties emerge. There may be differences not only between soluble and insoluble fiber, but among the various types of each. Some researchers believe that the distinction between fermentable and nonfermentable fiber will prove important.

The fiber furor is not likely to be settled for a long time, if at all. The only kind of study that *could* settle it would be a large-scale, prospective study on humans—something on the order of the famed Framingham (Massachusetts) study on cardiovascular disease, which has spanned decades and cost millions of dollars. No such study on fiber appears likely to be undertaken.

CAUTIOUS OPTIMISM ABOUT THE BENEFITS OF FIBER

After weighing the evidence on both sides of the controversy, scientists who are keeping close tabs on fiber research tend to be cautiously optimistic that appropriate fiber intake may indeed help to lessen people's chances of developing colon cancer. "There *is* something there," David Kritchevsky, associate director of Philadelphia's Wistar Institute and a prominent fiber researcher, told CU. The evidence, he said, favors the conclusion that insoluble dietary fiber offers some protection against colon cancer, though "it is much too early to be jumping to conclusions." He thinks the National Cancer Institute is pushing fiber too heavily, and he warns that some kinds of insoluble fiber actually increase the incidence of cancer in rats. In feeding rats increasingly large amounts of purified wood cellulose, he has observed an increasingly high incidence of cancer. He believes that mixtures of fiber, such as may be found in a varied diet, may offer the best protection.

Other researchers voice similar ideas. Peter Van Soest, professor of animal nutrition at Cornell University, stressed that both purified wood cellulose, and other finely ground types of fiber added to certain processed foods may do no good at all. Such highly refined fibers are broken into tiny particles that do not behave in the intestine the way the larger particles of unrefined fibers do. Coarsely ground bran, for instance, is an effective laxative, but finely ground bran can cause constipation. If you choose to sprinkle a bran supplement on top of your cereal or other foods, then it may be preferable to use one that's fairly coarse, not one that's ground to a powder.

Pending further research, we suggest that people increase consumption of foods containing fiber—both soluble and insoluble—rather than take fiber supplements. Eating more high-fiber foods is also likely to mean eating less fat—another beneficial measure.

HOW MUCH FIBER SHOULD YOU EAT?

The National Cancer Institute recommends a daily fiber intake of between 20 and 35 grams, depending on body weight. That's roughly double the amount of fiber the average American now consumes. CU's medical consultants think that's an appropriate range, but in the light of present knowledge would aim for the lower end of that range. The risk of side effects increases as you approach the upper end. Fiber consumption should not exceed 35 grams.

Rapidly adding fiber to the diet may have some side effects. A sudden, large increase in fiber intake can lead to bloating, flatulence, cramps, and diarrhea. You can avoid or minimize those side effects by adding fiber to the diet gradually.

Intestinal blockage can be caused by excessive fiber ingestion. In addition, heavy fiber intake may interfere with the absorption of minerals such as iron, copper, calcium, zinc, and magnesium. However, most researchers seem to agree that as long as people do not consume excessive levels of dietary fiber, and as long as they consume a balanced diet, they need not worry about fiber causing mineral imbalance or intestinal blockage.

Kellogg would have you get your fiber from *All-Bran*. The California Prune Board pushes its favorite product as "the high-fiber fruit," saying in ads that prunes have nine grams of fiber per six-prune serving—more fiber than in two servings of many bran cereals. But comparing sources of soluble and insoluble fiber is like comparing apples and oranges (or, more nearly, apples and bread). More neutral authorities believe that relying on just one fiber source might be hazardous, and recommend that you get your fiber from a variety of foods, such as those listed on page 116. We agree. As long as you don't overdo it, increasing your fiber intake probably can't hurt, and it may help.

12

Fear of Fat:
The Medical Evidence

At any given time, millions of Americans are dieting. Why? Mainly for appearance' sake—to fit, without bulging, into a culture that worships the svelte and trim. But there may be a more cogent reason for shedding pounds: to improve health and live longer.

In 1985, a panel convened by the National Institutes of Health (NIH) declared that obesity is a disease and a potential killer. The panel deplored what might be termed "the rounding of America." The nation now has a "high prevalence" of obesity among adults, the panelists said. And the increasing incidence of obesity in childhood and adolescence, they warned, will result in greater numbers of obese adults in the future.

Anyone 20 percent or more overweight—now the standard definition of obesity—should try to reduce, the NIH panel urged. That advice, it said, applied to 34 million obese Americans, or one out of every five adults. For some people, the panel said, even five excess pounds can threaten health.

At the same time, the panel's chairman, Jules Hirsch, M.D., of Rockefeller University, acknowledged that his group relied primarily on a "feeling for the data" in citing the figure of 20 percent above standard weight as the point at which a person ought to reduce. That's because hard information about the nature and consequences of obesity is still skimpy. Nor is there any consensus yet about just what is a person's "desirable weight."

HOW MUCH SHOULD YOU WEIGH?

To find out their ideal weight, Americans for more than 40 years have turned to the height/weight tables published by the Metropolitan Life Insurance Co.

The most recent Metropolitan desirable-weight tables, published in 1983, use combined data from 25 insurance companies that followed more than 4 million policyholders for between one and 22 years. The tables (pages 124–25) show the range of weights that were associated with lowest mortality among the policyholders. The weights shown are based on what people weighed at the time their insurance policies were issued. No attempt was made to monitor their changing weight as the years passed.

The NIH panel relied on the Metropolitan Life data, plus several other studies, in concluding that "obesity . . . has an adverse effect on longevity." In defining obesity, the panel began with a concept of ideal weight—the midpoint of the Metropolitan tables' desirable weight range for a person with a medium frame. If you weigh 20 percent more than that, you are obese and should reduce, the panel declared.

Unfortunately, the Metropolitan Life weight tables are far from a perfect indicator. For one thing, weight alone doesn't always reflect obesity, which is a measure of body fatness. Muscular athletes, for example, may be well over normal weight but not at all obese.

The percentage of your body weight that is in the form of fat is a better indicator of obesity than weight alone. However, measuring the percentage of body fat requires specialized equipment. The most accurate method requires immersion in a tank of water, which is awkward and expensive. A moderately accurate technique involves using calipers to measure the thickness of certain fleshy areas. Physicians and patients customarily rely on straight weight as an indicator.

Most of the data in the Metropolitan weight tables comes from white middle-class males—not a representative sample of the general U.S. population. The tables apply to people aged 25 to 59 and therefore don't cover younger adults or the growing number of people over 60.

Perhaps most important, the Metropolitan tables make no allowance for aging. They assume that a 50-year-old man, for example, should weigh the same as he did at 20. And that may be a mistake.

Reubin Andres, clinical director of the Gerontology Research Center at the National Institute on Aging, analyzed the insurance data from which Metropolitan Life derived its tables and found that the desirable weight-for-height varied markedly with age. He then devised a new weight table providing weight ranges associated with lowest mortality by age group.

BODY WEIGHTS

Height: Ft. and In. [1]	Metropolitan Life: Recommended Weights [1]		Gerontology Research Center: Age-Specific Weight Range for Men and Women					NIH Panel: Weight Indicating Obesity	
	Men	Women	20–29 yr.	30–39 yr.	40–49 yr.	50–59 yr.	60–69 yr.	Men	Women
4'10"	—	100–131	84–111	92–119	99–127	107–135	115–142	—	137
4'11"	—	101–134	87–115	95–123	103–131	111–139	119–147	—	139
5'0"	—	103–137	90–119	98–127	106–135	114–143	123–152	—	143
5'1"	123–145	105–140	93–123	101–131	110–140	118–148	127–157	157	146
5'2"	125–148	108–144	96–127	105–136	113–144	122–153	131–163	160	150
5'3"	127–151	111–148	99–131	108–140	117–149	126–158	135–168	162	154
5'4"	129–155	114–152	102–135	112–145	121–154	130–163	140–173	164	157

Height								
5'5"	131–159	117–156	106–140	115–149	125–159	134–168	144–179	167	161
5'6"	133–163	120–160	109–144	119–154	129–164	138–174	148–184	172	164
5'7"	135–167	123–164	112–148	122–159	133–169	143–179	153–190	175	168
5'8"	137–171	126–167	116–153	126–163	137–174	147–184	158–196	179	172
5'9"	139–175	129–170	119–157	130–168	141–179	151–190	162–201	182	175
5'10"	141–179	132–173	122–162	134–173	145–184	156–195	167–207	186	179
5'11"	144–183	135–176	126–167	137–178	149–190	160–201	172–213	190	182
6'0"	147–187	—	129–171	141–183	153–195	165–207	177–219	194	—
6'1"	150–192	—	133–176	145–188	157–200	169–213	182–225	199	—
6'2"	153–197	—	137–181	149–194	162–206	174–219	187–232	203	—
6'3"	157–202	—	141–186	153–199	166–212	179–225	192–238	211	—
6'4"	—	—	144–191	157–205	171–218	184–231	197–244	—	—

① Values in this table are for height without shoes and weight without clothes.

Remarkably, he found that the desirable weights for men and women of a given age and height were about the same.

Compared to the Metropolitan tables, Andres's table "permits" heavier weights for the middle-aged and elderly—but it's more restrictive for young people. The message of Andres's table is that average healthy individuals who are not overweight early in adulthood should not worry about putting on some extra pounds as they move into middle age. Andres has pointed to more than a dozen other studies also suggesting that middle-aged and older people live longer at weights the Metropolitan tables would consider too high.

Weight gain with age is certainly common in this country. Can some weight gain also be beneficial, as Andres contends? The NIH panel didn't think so. The panel mentioned Andres's work in its report but endorsed the Metropolitan tables as a guide for calculating desirable weights. However, a significant minority of obesity experts believe that the Metropolitan tables are too restrictive when they are applied to older people.

OBESITY AND HEALTH RISKS

When medical scientists speak of obesity raising the risk of mortality, they're mainly referring to the association between obesity and heart disease—the leading killer of Americans. It's not clear whether obesity per se directly promotes heart disease. What is certain is that obesity makes it much more likely that proven risk factors for heart disease will be present. Weight-related risk factors include hypertension (high blood pressure), high blood cholesterol levels, and diabetes. The NIH panel cited the following figures:

- Hypertension occurs about three times as often in overweight people as in those who are not overweight. Among adults aged 20 through 44, individuals 20 percent or more overweight are 5.6 times as likely as others to have hypertension.
- High blood cholesterol levels occur more than twice as often in overweight people.
- The prevalence of diabetes is nearly three times as high in the overweight.

Many studies have shown that weight loss can significantly improve all three of those heart-disease risk factors. If you're overweight and you have any of these risk factors or a family history of them, then losing weight should be a priority. Maintaining proper weight seems to be especially important for young males, obesity experts agree.

Recent evidence from several countries also suggests that *where* you're fat may be more important than how fat you are. So-called male-type obesity—the bulging abdomen sometimes known as beer belly or executive spread—seems to pose more of a threat than fat lower down around the hips and buttocks ("female type" obesity). Bulging bellies appear to increase the risk of developing cardiovascular disease and diabetes. Risk seems to increase sharply when the waist-to-hip ratio exceeds 1.0 in men and 0.8 in women. (In other words, men are at risk when their waist is larger than their hips; women are at risk when their waist measures more than 80 percent of their hips).

Why is abdominal fat worse? Researchers speculate that fat cells there may be more metabolically active, perhaps pumping more fat into the bloodstream and onto the artery walls.

Most of the population studies that have linked obesity to heart disease have focused on men, since they're much more likely to develop heart disease than women are. While obese women may or may not face the same heart-disease threat as men, they do face a cancer risk. Compared to nonoverweight women, obese women have a greater incidence of cancer of the gallbladder, uterus (including both cervix and endometrium), and ovaries. Postmenopausal obese women also have a heightened risk of breast cancer. Researchers believe that the uterine and breast cancers in obese women may result from the higher estrogen levels resulting from their obesity (fat stores can convert certain male adrenal hormones into female hormones). On the other hand, postmenopausal osteoporosis occurs less often among the obese for this same reason.

Obesity is also associated with several types of cancer in men: cancer of the colon, rectum, and prostate. Gallstone formation occurs much more often in obese people—especially women—than in others. The prevalence of arthritis and gout is also high among the obese.

Beyond its physiological effects, obesity can cause embarrassment and humiliation. The NIH panel even went so far as to say that the psychological burden of obesity may be "its greatest adverse effect."

While better health and greater longevity might be the reward of normal weight, the road there from obesity is paved with difficulties and potential health hazards of its own.

DIETS AND EXERCISE

About 30 years ago, an authority on the treatment of obesity had this to say: "Most obese persons will not stay in treatment of obesity. Of those who stay in treatment most will not lose weight and of those who do lose weight, most will regain it." The evidence behind that pessimistic assessment hasn't changed much. The problem facing dieters can be summed up this way: Losing weight is hard, but keeping it off is much harder.

There are complex and unresolved disputes about why people become overweight and remain that way despite strenuous efforts to reduce. Most experts believe that obesity results from an interaction among many factors—genetic, social, psychological, environmental, and hormonal. A number of explanations have been offered for how obesity occurs. Two hypotheses currently receiving a good deal of attention are the fat-cell theory and the set-point theory.

The fat-cell theory of obesity holds that a high-calorie diet in childhood leads the body to produce excessive numbers of fat cells, which a person then carries for life. Diet and exercise can help shrink these fat cells. But studies show that the number of fat cells can't be diminished—though they can still increase, especially in cases of extreme obesity.

According to the set-point theory of obesity, each of us is "programmed" to maintain a certain weight—much as a home's temperature is regulated by a thermostat. What we regard as an attempt to lose weight our body regards as famine—and responds accordingly. Shrunken fat cells, crying out to be filled, urge us to eat more. The body further defends its "set point" weight by lowering its metabolic rate, the rate at which energy is used by normal bodily processes. If valid, the set-point theory may help explain why diets often fail. After a person has shed a few pounds, losing weight becomes increasingly difficult, requiring more drastic calorie reductions. However, some proponents of the set-point theory believe that vigorous exercise can alter the body's "set point."

Regardless of the mechanism of obesity, resorting to fad and crash diets can cause serious illness and even death. Even ordinary dieting can cause frustration and depression. Weight-loss drugs can cause serious side effects. And the all-too-common "yo-yo" cycle of weight loss followed by weight gain may leave you worse off than before.

Some studies, mainly involving test animals, suggest that yo-yoing may actually cause some of the health problems that are blamed on obesity itself. In addition, people may regain increasingly more weight in successive cycles—and studies suggest that the regained weight contains an increasingly higher percentage of fat.

Since losing weight and keeping it off is so difficult, the best approach to managing obesity is to avoid it in the first place. People who really want to lose weight must forget about "going on a diet." Instead, they must undertake a permanent change in eating and living habits.

Your weight reflects the balance between calories ingested and calories expended. But many people still believe that overweight results solely from overeating. So when trying to lose weight, they usually limit themselves to dieting, and fail to achieve the desired result. Studies indicate that combining exercise with dieting may be the most effective way to lose weight and keep it off. As one report put it, overweight people can be thought of as underexercised rather than overfed.

Some people believe—mistakenly—that exercise increases appetite, making it even harder to limit eating. Actually, moderate exercise usually has very little effect on appetite.

Others contend that the modest calorie loss through exercise isn't worth the effort. Take jogging, they say: If one hour of jogging burns up only 500 calories, you need to jog for seven hours to lose one pound of body fat (3500 calories). That's true. But it's also true that jogging one-half hour a day for two weeks gives you those seven hours—and a one-pound loss. By jogging one-half hour per day for one year, while keeping food intake constant, you'd shed 26 pounds—far more than most crash diets promise, let alone deliver.

Ideally, when you diet you should lose fat, not muscle. Without exercise, you'll lose both. Dieters who also exercise lose weight mostly as fat.

If you're overweight, exercise can help you be healthier even if your caloric intake keeps you at the same weight. Besides improving muscle tone, exercise appears to help in reducing high blood pressure, lowering blood cholesterol levels, and improving blood sugar levels in diabetics, even when no weight loss occurs. Those changes, in turn, reduce the risk of heart disease.

13

Is There a Safe Sweetener?

Concerned about weight control and fearful of obesity, Americans have turned in increasing numbers to "diet" foods and beverages made with low-calorie artificial sweeteners—first cyclamate, then saccharin, then aspartame, and most recently acesulfame K. But the widespread use of artificial sweeteners has brought with it a raft of health concerns. People are still asking, "Is any sweetener safe?"

Thoughtful scientists generally address safety questions as a trade-off between risks and benefits. So far, any health benefit from artificial sweeteners remains largely a matter of conjecture. One might assume that artificial sweeteners are useful for weight control. But some authorities suggest that many people who use artificial sweeteners tend to increase their food consumption, leaving total calorie intake roughly unchanged or even increased. For some people, that diet soda may be a license for a slice of cake.

Surprisingly few studies have been undertaken to see whether artificial sweeteners actually help people control weight, and those few have been inconclusive. For example, the National Academy of Sciences/National Research Council assessed five studies concerning the "management of obesity with non-nutritive sweeteners." It found the design for all five studies "inappropriate" for reaching any firm conclusion on the efficacy of sweeteners in weight control.

Still, many people crave an alternative to sugar. For the nation's more than 11 million diabetics, that desire is especially compelling.

WHAT'S WRONG WITH SUGAR?

The average American consumes 67 pounds of assorted sugars per year. About half is sucrose, or table sugar. Most of the rest is made up of corn sweeteners, which are popular with food and beverage companies because they're cheap. But in calorie content, sucrose, corn sweeteners, and other sugars are equivalent. A teaspoon of sugar contains 16 calories, a can of sugar-sweetened soda, about 160.

Sugar is a natural suspect in obesity. Many grams of sugar fit into a small space; hence, candy and other sugar-laden foods pack a heavy load of calories. These carbohydrate calories are "empty," in that simple sugars provide only calories and no other nutrients to the body.

Weight gain results when one eats more calories—in any form—than one burns in exercising and carrying out normal activities. If you're trying to control your weight, sugar is only part of the picture. Fats have nine calories per gram, compared with four for sugar and other carbohydrates. But cutting down on consumption of simple sugars can certainly contribute to weight control.

Sugar has long been associated with tooth decay. Laboratory experiments have shown that forms of sugar that cling to the teeth—such as candy, honey, granulated sugar, and the like—are more damaging than the liquid forms, such as sugared beverages.

Among other charges leveled against sugar are that it promotes heart disease and that excessive sugar consumption may cause diabetes. An extensive review by the FDA recently concluded that there was no scientific basis for such assertions.

Though people with diabetes should watch their consumption of sugar, there is no evidence that excess sugar consumption causes diabetes. If sugar plays any role at all, it is an indirect one; it may contribute to obesity, which can in turn trigger the onset of diabetes in susceptible individuals. As for heart disease, any connection with sugar consumption remains speculative and unproved.

Overall, we see little harm in moderate sugar consumption.

CYCLAMATE: BANNED BUT NOT FORGOTTEN

Cyclamate *(Sucaryl)*, which is 30 times sweeter than an equal weight of sugar but calorie-free, was the dominant artificial sweetener in this country in the 1960s. Then tests with laboratory animals raised the possibility that it might cause cancer. The U.S. Food and Drug Administration (FDA) banned the use of cyclamate as a food additive in 1969. But it continues to be sold over-the-counter in drugstores in Canada and is also used in some 40 other countries.

To test the safety of a food additive, large doses are fed to small groups of animals. If it produces cancer or other toxic effects under laboratory conditions, the substance is presumed to pose some risk of causing similar effects in humans if very large numbers of users are exposed to low doses over many years. Direct evidence that a food additive causes adverse health effects in people is almost impossible to obtain, because people's eating habits are so complex and so many other variables influence people's health. Thus, animal data are usually the best evidence the FDA has available when evaluating the safety of an additive.

Though humans don't usually consume enormous doses of artificial sweeteners, many people do consume small amounts, day after day, year after year. And since nearly 70 million Americans use artificial sweeteners in one form or another, even a small risk could threaten a large number of people.

The initial evidence of cyclamate's possible health risks seemed damning at the time. In recent years, however, many scientists, manufacturers, and food and beverage companies have talked of getting the FDA to rescind its ban on cyclamate. The second thoughts arise out of a reevaluation of the original data, as well as more recent studies.

In 1984, the FDA's Cancer Assessment Committee reported on its review of more than two dozen studies on laboratory animals—mice, rats, dogs, and monkeys—that had been fed cyclamate for long periods. The committee said that some results could not be duplicated even by the authors of the studies and concluded that those studies showing a carcinogenic effect for the substance were open to question. It also said that "there is very little credible data to implicate cyclamate as a carcinogen at any organ tissue site. . . . "

On the strength of such reassessments, the makers of cyclamate, Abbott Laboratories, and a trade organization called the Calorie Control Council have petitioned the FDA to lift its ban on cyclamate.

Nevertheless, reasons for concern about other potential health effects of cyclamate remain. Various experiments have shown that a breakdown product of cyclamate, called cyclohexylamine (CHA), can cause high blood pressure and atrophy (shrinkage) of the testicles in rats.

In 1985, a committee of the National Academy of Sciences/National Research Council reviewed all the data assembled to date. It concluded that cyclamate and CHA are probably not carcinogens by themselves. It found the evidence "suggestive," however, that those substances may promote the effects of other cancer-causing substances or cause mutations. The committee also said that such other adverse side effects as testicular atrophy and toxicity to embryos must be fully investigated before cyclamate can be restored to use in the nation's food supply.

SACCHARIN: THE ENDLESS MORATORIUM

Some 300 times sweeter than sugar, and calorie-free, saccharin had taken over from cyclamate as the most commonly used artificial sweetener even before cyclamate was banned.

Numerous studies over the years have shown that saccharin is a weak carcinogen in laboratory animals. Rats fed large doses of saccharin showed an increased incidence of bladder cancer. The most influential of the many studies to date, a 1977 Canadian study, demonstrated that it was saccharin itself, not a contaminant or other factor, that produced cancer in test animals. In large part, it was this study that led the FDA in 1977 to propose banning saccharin in the U.S.

However, since cyclamate had already been banned in 1969, a ban on saccharin would have left the marketplace devoid of artificial sweeteners. A public outcry, eagerly fanned by the soft-drink industry, ensued. Congress, listening to the protests, imposed a moratorium on the saccharin ban. It has extended the moratorium every few years since.

Proponents of saccharin, including saccharin's only U.S. manufacturer, the Sherwin-Williams Company, note that people have been using saccharin for most of a century with no clear indication of ill effects, such as an increased incidence of bladder cancer in users. However, that does not necessarily mean that saccharin is without harm to humans.

Late in 1977, researchers at Johns Hopkins School of Medicine reported that pure saccharin did not cause genetic mutations in bacteria. (Many substances that cause such mutations are carcinogens, and most carcinogens cause mutations.) But the urine of mice fed saccharin did cause bacterial mutations, which suggests that a breakdown product of saccharin may be carcinogenic.

In 1978, Melvin Reuber, of the National Cancer Institute's Chemical Carcinogenesis Program, summarized many animal studies to date. He found that bladder cancer was not the only problem with saccharin. Various animal studies had reported cancers in the reproductive and blood-forming systems, in the lungs, and elsewhere. Reuber's judgment was that saccharin "likely is carcinogenic in human beings."

In 1983, Japanese researchers confirmed that saccharin promotes the action of a known carcinogen on the urinary bladder in rats. This finding added strength to previous evidence that saccharin, even if it is not cancer-causing in itself, may heighten the risk from substances that are. Such cancer promoters are called "co-carcinogens."

Also in 1983, the FDA's Frank Cordle and Sanford Miller said that even though saccharin is a known carcinogen and co-carcinogen in rodents, "the results of human epidemiologic studies tend to support the conclusion that human users of artificial sweeteners—saccharin and cyclamate—do not have an increased risk of cancer of the lower urinary tract." Cordle has said that he "would see very little hazard with humans" from exposure to saccharin and cyclamate.

But other scientists, including some on a National Research Council committee, find Cordle's assessment too optimistic. They point out that consumption of artificial sweeteners was relatively low until the last 20 years or so, and that many forms of cancer have a long latency period. Though no one has produced any proof that saccharin has been responsible for human cancer cases, at least one study has found that it can boost or promote the effects of known carcinogens on human cells in the test tube. Saccharin thus is a definite carcinogen in certain lab animals and may pose some risk as a carcinogen or co-carcinogen in humans. Research continues.

ASPARTAME: THE CHALLENGER

Aspartame *(Nutrasweet)* is a chemical combination of two amino acids, aspartic acid and phenylalanine. Both substances are building blocks of ordinary proteins and are essential nutrients. The FDA approved aspartame for certain uses in 1981 and for use in soft drinks in 1983.

Per gram, aspartame has just as many calories as sugar. However, since it is roughly 200 times sweeter than sugar, it contributes only ½₀₀ as many calories to the diet. Some aspartame preparations, such as the table-top sweetener *Equal,* use glucose as a carrier for the aspartame. That adds a few calories, but the total remains much lower than in an equivalent portion of sugar.

Toxicity tests have shown a short-term "no effect level" of 5000 milligrams per kilogram of body weight. That is, when test animals are given a single dose of up to 5000 milligrams (about a sixth of an ounce) of aspartame for every kilogram (2.2 pounds) they weigh, they show no signs of ill effects. The FDA has multiplied this figure by 100 as a safety factor and obtained a "maximum allowable daily intake" of 50 milligrams of aspartame per kilogram of body weight. That amounts to about 17 aspartame-sweetened sodas a day for a 150-pound adult, 8 or 9 such sodas for a 75-pound child.

The FDA has required aspartame's manufacturer, G.D. Searle, to monitor consumption levels. With the FDA's approval, Searle has contracted with the Market Research Corporation of America to survey users and calculate their levels of consumption of aspartame. Their reports show consumption levels for all age groups to be well within the FDA's limits. In assessing health hazards, the practice is to focus on the 1 percent of users who consume the largest quantities of the sweetener.

One of the two components of aspartame, phenylalanine, poses problems for some people—roughly one in 15,000—who suffer from a metabolic disorder called phenylketonuria (PKU). These people lack an enzyme needed to process this amino acid properly, which can build up to toxic levels in their blood and tissues. If the condition is not diagnosed at birth, mental retardation can result. Fortunately, screening at birth is now routine.

To make sure that people afflicted with PKU know of the phenylalanine in aspartame, the FDA requires that aspartame-containing products be labeled with a warning.

When aspartame breaks down, either before or after consumption, it releases a substance called diketopiperazine (DKP) and methyl alcohol. The latter is simple wood alcohol, famous for causing blindness and brain damage in drinkers of bootleg liquor and *Sterno.*

But early concern about the products of aspartame breakdown seems to have eased. The FDA concluded that at doses considerably above any likely dietary intake, DKP is not toxic to adults, children, or fetuses, and does not cause mutations in bacteria. As for methyl alcohol, many foods contain more of it than aspartame produces. The aspartame in one can of diet soda, for example, provides only about half as much methyl alcohol as eight ounces of tomato juice—and both sources contain much less than the body can process without ill effects.

Perhaps more worrisome have been concerns raised by John Olney, of Washington University in St. Louis, and Richard Wurtman, a professor of biochemistry at M.I.T. They have warned that, because aspartame's components are related to neurotransmitters—chemicals that pass signals from nerve cell to nerve cell—and since aspartic acid and phenylalanine levels in the blood do rise at least a little after a person consumes aspartame, the sweetener might adversely affect the brain.

The FDA, after an analysis of Dr. Wurtman's studies and others, disagreed with his conclusions, saying that the evidence for behavioral effects is not significant and that no further behavioral testing seems necessary. The British government has reached a similar conclusion.

In 1983, the FDA said that it is reasonably certain that aspartame does not cause brain tumors, brain damage, or behavioral changes in humans.

But Wurtman, despite all signs of safety, has maintained that the FDA showed "unseemly haste" in approving aspartame. Florence Graves, as vice president of Common Cause, has expressed the same concern. She has stated that aspartame was approved for use in soft drinks in large part because of the antiregulatory stance of the Reagan administration—and perhaps because of a wish to reduce saccharin consumption by providing an alternative.

The FDA began monitoring the growing number of complaints from consumers about possible side effects of aspartame use. In 1984, the FDA asked the Centers for Disease Control (CDC) for help in analyzing and evaluating these complaints. By the end of the year, the CDC said that the reported symptoms—including stomach upset, hives, headaches, menstrual problems, insomnia, and uncontrollable behavior—fit no specific pattern. Furthermore, the CDC said, the symptoms were generally mild, common even among people who did not use aspartame, and most abundant in Arizona, where adverse publicity had been especially prominent. The CDC's position is that while some people may be unusually sensitive to aspartame, the data "do not provide evidence for the existence of serious, widespread, adverse health consequences," especially since similar complaints have not surfaced in other countries where aspartame is being used. The CDC's report also stated that a thorough evaluation of the complaints would require "focused clinical studies," several of which are now planned or under way.

Despite the uncertainty, aspartame received an impressive endorsement in 1985. The Council on Scientific Affairs of the American Medical Association stated: "Available evidence suggests that consumption of aspartame by normal humans is safe and is not associated with serious adverse health effects. Individuals who need to control their phenylalanine intake should handle aspartame like any other source of phenylalanine."

ACESULFAME K: THE LATEST ENTRY

A new artificial sweetener entered the U.S. marketplace more recently, having previously been used in 20 countries, including Australia, Britain, France, Israel, Sweden, Switzerland, the Soviet Union, and West Germany. In 1988, the FDA approved acesulfame potassium—or acesulfame K—as a table sugar substitute and for use in dry food products. The manufacturer expects to win approval for use in liquids, baked goods, candies, and, ultimately, soft drinks. The sweetener is marketed in the United States under the brand name *Sunette.*

Acesulfame K, like aspartame, is about 200 times sweeter than sugar. Like saccharin, it has no calories. Acesulfame K's reported advantages over the other two include greater stability, lack of an aftertaste, and lower cost.

But even before the product was approved by the FDA, its safety had been challenged by the Center for Science in the Public Interest, a nutrition-oriented consumer advocacy group that has often challenged the safety of artificial sweeteners. The organization asserted that some studies showed an increased incidence of tumors and a rise in blood cholesterol among laboratory animals that were fed the sweetener. The FDA, however, concluded that the animals' health problems "were typical of what could routinely be expected and were not due to feeding with acesulfame potassium."

Clearly, the acesulfame K story has only just begun.

RECOMMENDATIONS

With the exception of diabetics, few people really *need* artificial sweeteners. Sugar, used in moderation, has no serious adverse health effects, and it has fewer calories than some people assume.

Saccharin's demonstrated carcinogenicity in laboratory animals is a serious problem, in CU's view. We believe that Congress should rescind its moratorium and let the FDA make an independent decision about saccharin, which it proposed to ban in 1977.

A reexamination of the evidence suggests that cyclamate is not itself a carcinogen and has no adverse effect on brain function. However, there remain unresolved concerns about its overall safety, including whether it may act as a co-carcinogen to promote the effects of some known carcinogens. In addition, since it is only 30 times as sweet as sugar, it is harder to keep its consumption down to levels presumed safe. We think there are too many unresolved questions to put cyclamate back on the market.

Although some questions remain about aspartame's safety, and about the soundness of the process that led to its approval, it seems to be acceptably safe for most people when used in moderation. It does not appear to cause or promote cancer. But it may, as the label warns, pose a potential risk for people with PKU. For the time being, an objective weighing of the evidence suggests that aspartame is the artificial sweetener to be preferred on safety grounds.

As of this writing, it is still too early to reach firm conclusions about the long-term safety of the just-approved acesulfame K.

On the road to ideal weight, sugar-free products can take you only so far. To go the distance, you'll have to rely on a carefully planned, and persistent, regimen that provides fewer total calories and more vigorous exercise. (For details, see Chapter 12, "Fear of Fat.")

14

The Vitamin Pushers

In 1936, CU published a report called "The Vitamin Stampede," which deplored the overselling of vitamins to the U.S. population. The report lamented that vitamins were being "forced on children and adults without sufficient thought and understanding."

At that time, some experiments had suggested that a certain vitamin might help to prevent colds. But more careful and controlled trials had indicated, as the 1936 report put it, "that [this substance] cannot be counted on to influence respiratory infections." Vitamin C? No, it was vitamin A back then.

Today, the buzzwords for selling vitamins have been modernized—though vitamins themselves, and the human body's limited need for them, have remained the same. A recent trend is to push vitamins for the relief of "stress." Almost everyone, of course, experiences stress. If it follows that almost everyone needs vitamin supplements, commercial logic is satisfied—if not the scientific method.

In 1985, the U.S. Food and Drug Administration (FDA) and the Pharmaceutical Advertising Council began a major campaign of public-service ads attacking quackery and encouraging people to ask their physician or pharmacist about claims that seem too good to be true. Curious about what advice pharmacists give their customers about vitamins, CU sent reporters, posing as customers, to 30 pharmacies in Pennsylvania, Missouri, and California.

Our customers told the pharmacists that they'd been feeling nervous or tired lately, and asked whether a vitamin would help. In fact, neither nervousness nor fatigue calls for vitamin supplementation. But most of the 30 pharmacists seemed more than willing to sell vitamin pills for those purposes. Only nine mentioned the possibility of seeing a physician.

Pharmacists are only one part of the picture. Drug-company advertising is another big part. Pushed by the ads, the public has developed quite an appetite for vitamin pills—as well as for many other types of "dietary supplements" (see Chapter 25). Surveys suggest that about half of all

Americans take a vitamin pill either regularly or occasionally—and some people take a handful or more every day.

Most vitamin users, concerned that their diet may not be adequate, take their daily doses as "insurance" against deficiency. Others—operating on the dangerously mistaken theory that if some is good, more must be better—hope that the products will provide extra energy, prevent or cure disease, protect against stress, or enhance athletic ability.

WHAT VITAMINS ARE—AND HOW MUCH YOU REALLY NEED

A vitamin is an organic substance required to promote one or more essential biochemical reactions within living cells. Unlike foods, vitamins are needed only in tiny amounts and are not a source of energy (calories). For a substance to qualify as a vitamin, its absence must cause a specific deficiency disease that is cured when the substance is resupplied. (Lack of vitamin C, for example, causes scurvy, which can be cured with vitamin C.)

There are 13 known vitamins required by humans. Four are fat-soluble (A, D, E, and K), and nine are water-soluble (C and the eight "B-complex" vitamins—thiamin, riboflavin, niacin, B_6, folic acid, B_{12}, pantothenic acid, and biotin). Do any more remain to be discovered? Probably not, since patients have survived for years on intravenous feedings fortified with only these vitamins. Hucksters continue to tout non-vitamin substances such as P, B_{15}, and B_{17} as vitamins, but they are not and never will be.

The Food and Nutrition Board of the National Academy of Sciences/National Research Council publishes guidelines known as the Recommended Dietary Allowances (RDAs) for essential nutrients—protein, carbohydrates, fat, minerals, and vitamins. The RDAs are defined as "the levels of intake of essential nutrients considered adequate to meet the known nutritional needs of practically all healthy persons."

These are not "minimums" or "requirements." The level for each nutrient is deliberately set higher than most people need. The RDA for each vitamin is usually derived by estimating the range of normal human needs, selecting the number at the high end of that range, and adding a safety factor. The values vary somewhat by age and sex, and are increased for women during pregnancy and breast-feeding.

For three vitamins—K, pantothenic acid, and biotin—the Food and Nutrition Board has published "estimated safe and adequate intakes" rather than RDAs. This was done because part of people's need for those vitamins is supplied by bacteria within the intestines; how much must come from food is not known.

The FDA took the National Research Council's figures and simplified them to create the U.S. Recommended Daily Allowances (U.S. RDAs), which you see on many food labels. U.S. RDAs generally represent the highest level of the National Research Council's RDAs for each nutrient. Therefore, few if any people need more than the U.S. RDAs. Most people can do just fine on less. (In our discussion, RDA refers to the National Research Council's Recommended Dietary Allowances.)

FALSE ALARMS ABOUT NUTRITIONAL DEFICIENCIES

Many vitamin enthusiasts suggest that everyone should take supplements to be sure of getting enough. They say, for example, that "eating on the run" and "overprocessing" of foods place the typical American in danger of deficiency. Some also speak of "soil depletion" and dieting as reasons why people need vitamin supplements.

Such arguments amount to false alarms.

It's true that many Americans commonly eat on the run, skip entire meals, and watch their weight. But it's unlikely that those habits are breeding vitamin deficiencies.

Fast-food meals, for instance, can be reasonably nutritious, especially if you patronize the salad bar. The main problem with fast food is not what's missing but what's present—a lot of calories, sodium, and fat.

As for skipping meals, many people do, but those who eat only one or two meals daily during the week usually more than make up for any deficits with snacks and with increased variety and abundance on weekends.

Dieting should be done sensibly, of course (see Chapter 12). But only prolonged or highly unbalanced diets (such as very low calorie diets or macrobiotic diets) could create a risk of vitamin deficiency.

The argument about "overprocessing" of foods oversimplifies a complex issue. Processing can remove some vitamins and other nutrients, but it can also restore them or add missing ones.

Our consultants scoff at the idea that depleted soil robs the American diet of vitamins. A plant's mineral content may be influenced somewhat by soil composition, but its vitamin content is largely determined by the plant's heredity. A carrot grown in depleted soil, for instance, may be stunted—but its vitamin A content (per unit weight) will be the same as if it had been grown in enriched soil.

Finally, some vitamins are lost in cooking. But losses of that sort are usually only partial, and are compensated for by including uncooked fruits and vegetables in your diet.

The suggestion to buy "nutrition insurance" in pill form can be very appealing, and vitamin manufacturers have run ad campaigns to promote use of their products for that purpose.

But nutrition authorities question the need for such supplements. According to Victor Herbert, professor of medicine at Mount Sinai School of Medicine in New York City, "Vitamin pushers use deception by omission. They list all the terrible things that can happen if your diet is lacking. But they never tell you that vitamin deficiency is rare unless a person's diet is extremely unbalanced. Most important, they never tell how to measure whether or not your diet is adequate. If they did, they'd lose customers. Determining dietary adequacy is actually quite easy."

You can get an adequate amount of all essential nutrients by planning your meals to include what nutritionists call the Basic Four Food Groups. Your average daily intake should include:

- Four servings of vegetables, fruits, and fruit juices, at least one of which should be fresh.
- Four servings of grain and cereal products (including cereals, breads, rice, macaroni, and the like).
- Two to four servings of meats or alternatives such as fish, poultry, eggs, or beans.
- Two to four servings of milk or dairy products.

Because foods within each group differ in nutrient content, choosing a variety within each group is important. Adhering to the recommended number of servings, with reasonable portion sizes, would provide about 1200 calories and sufficient amounts of all essential nutrients. Since most people eat more than that, it should be clear that eating a wide variety of foods from the Basic Four will easily provide the nutrients you need. Further, though some advocates would lead you to believe otherwise, a few days without one vitamin or another will do you no real harm.

HYPE ABOUT STRESS

If the "nutrition insurance" appeal is old news, the new ploy in selling vitamins is to offer you protection against stress. Typical "stress formula" vitamin products contain 10 or more times the RDA for vitamin C and for several of the B vitamins. While some vitamin promoters refer only to physical stresses, others include mental stress, overwork, and the like. Some make no health claims at all, but rely on the word *stress* in the product's name to sell it.

According to Lederle Laboratories, makers of *Stresstabs 600,* the concept of high-dosage stress vitamins is based on a 1952 National Research Council report that recommended extra vitamins for people suffering from stresses such as general surgery, serious burns, and major fractures. However, the report explicitly stated that "in minor illnesses or injury where the expected duration of the disease is less than 10 days and when the patient is essentially ambulatory and is eating his diet . . . a good diet will supply the Recommended Dietary Allowances of all nutrients."

Nutrition experts advise that although vitamin needs may rise with certain physical conditions, they seldom rise above the Recommended Dietary Allowances—and are easily met by proper eating. Someone who is under enough stress to incur vitamin deficiency would probably be sick enough to be in a hospital. But ads for "stress vitamins" have generally been aimed at well-nourished members of the general public.

No evidence exists that *emotional* stress increases the body's need for vitamins.

HYPE FOR ATHLETES AND SMOKERS

Athletes, from the professional to the weekend jogger, may be tempted to pop vitamin pills to achieve better performance or to replenish vitamins lost through vigorous activity.

It is true that strenuous exercise increases the need for calories, water, and a few nutrients. However, vitamin needs are unlikely to rise above the RDA amounts available from a balanced diet. The notion that extra vitamins are useful to athletes is also tied to the idea that extra vitamins provide extra energy—which is untrue. Energy comes from the calories in food, and vitamins have no caloric value.

A cascade of advertising hypes vitamins for athletes. Revco's *Competition Plus*—"for extra effort sports"—have claimed to "meet the special nutritional needs of sports active people."

Smokers are known to have lower blood levels of vitamin C than do nonsmokers, which has led some promoters to suggest that smokers should take extra vitamin C. But according to Victor Herbert, "There is no credible evidence that smokers need more than RDA amounts of vitamin C. The 1980 RDA amounts are at least four times as much as a normal person would ever need in a day."

Alfred E. Harper, professor of biochemistry and nutrition sciences at the University of Wisconsin, who chaired the 1974 National Research Council RDA Committee, says, "Since most subjects used in the major experiments that served as the basis for present vitamin C allowances were smokers, the suggestion that smokers need high doses of vitamin C seems incongruous. If anything, it would seem much more appropriate to suggest that nonsmokers need less."

OTHER POPULAR VITAMIN MYTHS

Vitamin C and Colds   Proponents of vitamin C—most notably the chemist and Nobel laureate Linus Pauling—claim that it can help prevent colds in daily doses of 1000 milligrams or more. But at least 16 double-blind studies over the past decade have found no such benefit.

The classic series of studies was conducted by researchers at the University of Toronto. They concluded that vitamin C did not prevent colds at all, but did help to reduce slightly the severity of certain cold symptoms. This mild benefit was achieved with a daily dose of 250 milligrams (about the amount in two 8-ounce glasses of orange juice). Higher doses provided no extra benefit. Indeed, the researchers eventually concluded that only 120 milligrams daily was enough.

Vitamin C and Cancer   Pauling and some others also believe that massive doses of vitamin C can prolong the life of cancer patients. This claim is based on a study he reported with Ewan Cameron, a Scottish physician. However, researchers who analyzed the report concluded that the study was not properly designed.

The Mayo Clinic has conducted two clinical trials to test the effectiveness of vitamin C and cancer, each involving 100 or more patients in the advanced stage of the disease. Half the patients received vitamin C, half a placebo. The researchers found no differences in survival time, appetite, severity of pain, weight loss, or amount of nausea and vomiting.

Vitamin E and Breast Lumps   Several years ago, preliminary studies by Robert London, M.D., and colleagues at Sinai Hospital of Baltimore suggested that vitamin E supplements might help women with mammary dysplasia (also called benign fibrocystic disease of the breast). But two well-designed, double-blind studies reported in 1985—including one by Dr. London's team—found no significant benefit.

B_6 for Premenstrual Syndrome   High dosages of vitamin B_6 have been widely advanced as a treatment for premenstrual syndrome. The evidence supporting this practice is thin—mixed results in small scale studies. Since most water-soluble vitamins are relatively safe in large doses (in contrast to fat-soluble vitamins, which are not), some physicians felt comfortable in recommending B_6 in the range of 200 to 800 milligrams daily. (That dose is 100 to 400 times the RDA.)

In recent years, however, physicians have reported seeing damage to the nervous system in individuals who took 500-milligram doses of B_6, and in one person whose reported intake was 200 milligrams a day for three years. Their symptoms, which resembled those of multiple sclerosis, included numbness and tingling of the hands, difficulty in walking, and the sensation of electric shocks shooting down the spine. In light of these cases, we advise against megadoses of vitamin B_6. CU's medical consultants take a dim view of megadose B_6 therapy because of possible peripheral nerve toxicity.

GENUINE NUTRITIONAL SHORTAGES

Although vitamin deficiencies are rare among people who eat a reasonably varied diet, a fair number of Americans may need more of certain minerals. Some people—especially women—should pay special attention to these three:

- **Calcium** deserves particular attention because inadequate calcium intake is a factor in the development of osteoporosis, or thinning of the bones, especially in women. Those who like milk, cheese, and other dairy products may get what they need from diet alone. But those consuming little calcium-rich food should seek advice on supplementation from a physician or registered dietician. (See Chapter 25.)
- **Iron** is needed to make hemoglobin, the component in red blood cells that carries oxygen to the tissues. Lack of sufficient iron causes iron-deficiency anemia. Women who are pregnant or who menstruate heavily should be checked by a physician to be sure they are not anemic and for advice on possible iron supplements.
- **Fluoride** intake throughout childhood helps build decay-resistant teeth. The most efficient, economical way to get it is through fluoridated water. Children who grow up in nonfluoridated communities should take supplementary fluoride (by prescription) from birth through age 12. (See Chapter 19.)

DANGERS OF EXCESS

Fat-soluble vitamins are not excreted efficiently. They are generally stored in the body until they can be used up, and thus can accumulate to toxic levels. For example, prolonged excessive intake of vitamin A can cause headache, increased pressure on the brain, bone pain, and damage to the liver. Excessive vitamin D can cause kidney stones and eventual kidney damage.

Though water-soluble vitamins are generally excreted in the urine when taken in excess, some of them can cause trouble. There's the risk of permanent damage to the nervous system resulting from sustained high doses of vitamin B_6, mentioned above. Large doses of niacin can cause severe flushes, skin rash, and abnormal liver-function tests. And high doses of vitamin C can cause diarrhea.

Reported cases of actual vitamin toxicity are uncommon. But they are particularly sad because most people who get into trouble with vitamins have essentially poisoned themselves in the pursuit of health.

RECOMMENDATIONS

The best way to get vitamins is from foods in a balanced diet. Vitamin supplementation may be appropriate for children up to two years, for older children who have poor eating habits, for some people on prolonged weight-reduction programs, for pregnant women, for strict vegetarians (those who avoid eggs and milk as well as meat), and for people with certain illnesses, as directed by a physician.

Rather than taking vitamins for "insurance," evaluate your diet to determine whether you are eating a variety of foods from the Basic Four groups. If you have trouble figuring that out by yourself, record what you eat for a week and ask a registered dietitian or a physician whether you are missing anything. If you are, the best course of action will probably be to improve your eating habits, not to take supplements.

As a rule, don't take more than the RDA amounts except on medical advice. And avoid doctors or nutrition consultants who recommend vitamins as a cure-all.

CU urges that several things be done to clean up the vitamin marketplace. The FDA should evaluate the claims made by promoters of vitamins and publicize its findings. It should also work with the pharmaceutical industry to develop voluntary standards for vitamin-product formulations. The Federal Trade Commission should attempt to stop misleading advertising related to vitamins. And the pharmaceutical profession should recognize the pushing of unnecessary supplements as an ethical issue that deserves its serious attention.

SKIN
and
HAIR

15

Acne

In a society where clean, smooth skin, free of blemishes, seems to be a prerequisite for social acceptance, acne can be a severe test of one's emotional stamina. It usually occurs during adolescence—precisely when increasing maturity is striving for expression, and appearance has assumed enormous importance. Young adults, particularly women, may also experience a distressing outbreak of acne where once there was none. (The abrupt onset of acne in middle age may be a symptom of an endocrine disorder that merits consultation with a physician.)

Although it is not a life-threatening disease and only occasionally results in disfiguring scars, acne often causes immeasurable mental anguish to those afflicted. Advertisers of skin preparations play on these anxieties in promoting their products. Some self-help products can indeed serve a useful function in acne care. But to understand why over-the-counter (OTC) medication is so problematical, one needs to understand the factors that lead to acne.

UNDERSTANDING ACNE

Acne (eruption of the face) *vulgaris* (common) is primarily a disorder of the so-called pilosebaceous units of certain areas of the skin. Each unit consists of a hair follicle—from which a hair shaft protrudes—and a sebaceous gland that secretes sebum (a whitish fatty substance) into the follicle and through the pores to the surface of the skin adjacent to the hair shaft. The normal follicle is lined with cells that age, die, and are easily extruded through the pores of the skin. In time, these cells are replaced by new cells and the cycle is repeated.

Acne is caused by an abnormality in this orderly process of cell extrusion and replacement. When the skin pore becomes blocked with cellular debris, sebum cannot escape through the blocked pore onto the skin surface. The primary lesions of acne that result are comedones (whiteheads): collections of dead cells, sebum, and bacteria that clog the shaft of the hair follicle. On exposure to air, comedones darken (blackheads).

Many dermatologists believe that, as the amount of sebum within the pilosebaceous unit increases, the follicle's normal bacteria release an enzyme that splits the sebum into smaller molecules called fatty acids. Acting as irritants, those fatty acids then cause disruption of the follicular wall—and additional lesions called papules and pustules appear. Papules are red, solid areas that protrude above the skin surface. Pustules are papules that extend deeper into the skin and contain pus. Most of us know these lesions as pimples.

The amount of sebum secreted varies widely in different areas of the skin. The most active sebaceous glands are located in the scalp, followed by the forehead, face, chest, and upper back. Except for the scalp, these areas are the most frequent sites of acne.

As part of the normal maturing process, the sebaceous glands at puberty increase in size and secrete more sebum under the influence of increasing amounts of sex hormones, principally the male hormone testosterone, present in both males and females. The increased sebum production, combined with obstruction of the pores by cellular debris, sets the stage for the development of acne. If the overactivity of the sebaceous glands or the plugging of the pores could be better controlled, acne might pose less of a problem.

OVER-THE-COUNTER MEDICATIONS

Unless acne is severe, a visit to the doctor is not usually necessary. Only about one case in 10 deserves medical attention. Most mild or moderate cases of acne respond to effective OTC medication and to home care.

An assortment of OTC acne products crowds the marketplace. Besides the creams, cleansers, lotions, soaps, powders, and gels you might expect, you can also buy cleansing sticks, scrubs, medicated towelettes, tablets, and many other items. Except for cosmetic agents designed solely to camouflage the lesions, many of these products contain the same time-worn medicaments tried by physicians through the years in an attempt to manage this stubborn disorder.

An advisory panel that reviewed OTC acne remedies for the U.S. Food and Drug Administration (FDA) found four common ingredients to be of value. Of these, the most effective by far is benzoyl peroxide, which forms the basis of many OTC products (such as *Benoxyl 10, Fostex, Loroxide, Noxzema Acne-12, Oxy-5, Oxy-10, Oxy-10 Wash,* and *Vanoxide*). The other three ingredients, sulfur, sulfur/resorcinol combined, and salicylic acid, were found to be safe and effective only in mild cases. The rationale for each of these ingredients is their irritative effect by which they tend to unplug follicles. Avoid OTC products that do not list at least one of these active ingredients on the label.

Because people differ in the sensitivity of their skin and the severity of their acne, no single acne product is ideal for everyone. If your skin is sensitive and your acne mild, try a product with a 5 percent concentration of benzoyl peroxide. If your skin is not especially sensitive and your acne moderate, you might start with a 10 percent benzoyl peroxide formulation. If either product seems unsuitable—too weak or too harsh—switch accordingly.

Follow directions carefully. If your skin becomes overly dry and scaly—even with a mild product—stop applications for a while and also cut down on your use of soap.

PRESCRIPTION MEDICATIONS

Acne patients whose skin has not responded to OTC medications may decide to consult a physician. And certainly all those with severe cases of acne should seek help to prevent destruction of tissue and to minimize the possibility of permanent scarring. If you do need medical help for acne, first consult your family physician, who can then decide whether to treat your case or to refer you to a dermatologist. A doctor can prescribe medication specifically tailored to each patient's needs, with dosage and proportion of ingredients adjusted individually. Acne usually can be kept under control until the passage of time obviates the need for treatment.

The anti-acne arsenal available to physicians also includes the injection of corticosteroids into acne cysts, cryotherapy, dermabrasion, tissue elevation, and incision and drainage of pustules. However, none of these treatments can eliminate acne.

Antibiotics, in usual therapeutic doses, have long been prescribed by physicians to treat particularly severe cases of acne. In recent years, physicians have found that smaller doses of broad-spectrum antibiotics, administered daily for months or even years, have had a beneficial effect on many patients with moderate acne. This low-dose antibiotic therapy has been shown to reduce the concentration of free fatty acids that irritate the hair follicle. Researchers believe that antibiotics achieve this effect by decreasing the number of bacteria in the follicle, thereby limiting the amount of bacterial enzymes that split the sebum into fatty acids. Barring allergic reactions, side effects from such low-dose antibiotic therapy are generally minimal, with gastrointestinal upset the most common complaint.

Antibiotics in special lotion or gel form have been developed that are at least as effective as low-dose oral antibiotics against moderate acne. Available by prescription, this topical form of treatment does not cause the side effects sometimes seen with oral antibiotics.

For severe acne, dermatologists frequently administer benzoyl peroxide in a gel form together with antibiotics—either oral or topical.

Tretinoin (vitamin A acid, trade name Retin-A) was approved by the FDA in 1972 as a topical prescription preparation. (Many people now know Retin-A as an antiwrinkle cream that is said to reverse the skin's aging response to sun exposure, discussed on pages 161–62). Available in gel, cream, and liquid forms, tretinoin appears to be particularly useful in clearing the follicle opening, thereby reducing the number of acne lesions. However, patience is required. Skin irritation is common at first; the acne may even appear to worsen during the first six weeks of treatment, and improvement is rarely seen before three months. CU's medical consultants advise pregnant women to avoid using tretinoin.

Some people treated with tretinoin also experience a photosensitivity reaction (an intense reaction to sunlight resulting in skin reddening and painful blistering) as well as mild loss of skin pigment. People using this medication should minimize their exposure to the sun and stay under the continued supervision of a dermatologist. Tretinoin is sometimes given together with benzoyl peroxide for an additive effect: tretinoin by night and benzoyl peroxide by day.

Besides this topical use of vitamin A acid, some people have advocated taking large oral doses of vitamin A supplements. In true vitamin A deficiency—which is extremely rare—the skin and the mucous membrane, including the lining of the hair follicle, become thickened and tough. Since acne involves similar changes in the hair follicle, some physicians have reasoned that megadoses of vitamin A may prevent or cure the condition. In most cases, however, the treatment has been unsuccessful.

In one large study, college students with acne were given 100,000 units of vitamin A a day—about 20 times the recommended daily allowance. Slightly more than half of them showed some improvement—but so did half of a control group that received only a placebo. Taking vitamin A in doses greater than 50,000 units a day for several months can cause a range of side effects, including loss of body hair, itchy skin, enlargement of the liver and spleen, and increased pressure inside the head.

Large doses of estrogen, the female sex hormone, have been prescribed for potentially disfiguring acne in women. The hormone works by reducing sebaceous gland secretions. Such therapy, however, may stunt growth and is therefore inadvisable in a still-growing female. And estrogen has become an uncommon anti-acne strategy since the introduction of Accutane.

Accutane: Savior or Scourge?

In 1982, a synthetic relative of vitamin A, isotretinoin (Accutane), was approved by the FDA for the "treatment of severe, recalcitrant, cystic acne unresponsive to conventional therapy, including systemic antibiotics." Hailed by *The Medical Letter* as "the most effective treatment ever offered for acne"—a statement seconded by the American Academy of Dermatology—the drug produces dramatic, nearly complete clearing of acne lesions in more than 80 percent of patients. The improvement is often permanent after four to five months of treatment.

Taken orally by prescription, Accutane produces a number of temporary side effects, and its use requires careful supervision by a physician. Nearly all patients experience chapped lips and dry, itchy skin, and many develop eye irritation. Some may also suffer from muscle or joint pains, headache, fatigue, rash, or gastrointestinal symptoms. Many of these side effects can be relieved by topical lubricants or other drugs, and all disappear when treatment is stopped. Long-term effects have not been established.

But the most serious problems with Accutane are severe and often lethal birth defects in children born to women who become pregnant while taking the drug. (Accutane does not harm a woman's gametes—the sex cells that pass on hereditary material—so later pregnancies are not affected by prior use of the drug.) Accutane's manufacturer, Hoffmann-La Roche, deserves credit for having swiftly launched an extensive educational campaign notifying physicians, pharmacists, and patients (through brochures and leaflets) about the birth-defect potential. As a result, many physicians have required that female patients take pregnancy tests before beginning Accutane therapy, and urged them to employ at least one birth-control method during treatment and for one month before and after.

The message did not reach far enough. Between 1982 and 1986, the number of babies born with defects caused by the drug was anywhere from 62 to 1300—depending on whether you accept the manufacturer's estimates (based on actual reported cases) or the FDA's (based on extrapolation from that data).

In the spring of 1988, an expert advisory committee to the FDA recommended that distribution of Accutane be severely restricted to make it more difficult for young women to obtain. Soon thereafter the FDA instituted requirements that women sign a consent form before being given a prescription for Accutane, and that Hoffmann-La Roche print a warning picture of a deformed baby on Accutane packaging to help drive the message home.

In midsummer of the same year, the American Academy of Dermatology mailed new guidelines to its members. The academy said there were now 69 reported cases of Accutane-associated birth defects since 1982. The guidelines recommended that women taking Accutane test negative for pregnancy within two weeks of starting the drug, and that they use effective methods of contraception, with monthly blood pregnancy tests, throughout the therapy and for a month thereafter. Women intending to become pregnant should stop taking Accutane at least three months before conception.

TREATING ACNE YOURSELF

In self-treatment of acne, dermatologists recommend that the face be washed two or three times daily with soap and warm water, and rinsed thoroughly. There is no actual proof that face washing helps. But gentle scrubbing with a soapy washcloth does remove some oils, dead skin, and surface bacteria. It also produces minor irritation, which may be of some help in mild acne.

In any case, success does not depend on the type of soap used. Such heavily advertised cleansing products as *Noxzema Medicated Skin Cream* and *Cuticura Medicated Soap* are no more useful than a bar of plain soap. "Acne soaps" with sulfur are not particularly helpful because the medication is likely to wash away with rinsing.

While antibacterial soaps are indeed effective in reducing the number of skin surface bacteria, they are irrelevant for acne therapy. Although bacteria are the source of the enzymes that break down sebum into troublesome free fatty acids, these bacteria live beneath the skin's surface, deep in the follicles. They cannot be reached by the antibacterial ingredients in OTC cleansing products.

Of limited value for some people are abrasive soaps, such as *Brasivol,* which contain irritating granules. These products physically induce inflammation, and can be quite harsh to sensitive skin.

Many women, influenced by cosmetic advertising, have developed the habit of using face creams in place of soap and water for cleansing the face. This is not wise for people with acne, because greases and creams encourage plugging of the pores. So-called skin foods, skin tonics, lubricating creams, and vanishing creams should be avoided, too.

Even though the desire to cover up blemishes may be overwhelming, it's best not to use any cosmetics. For those who can't resist, water-based products, applied lightly, are the least likely to cause problems. If the hair is naturally oily, it should be kept off the face. Hair dressings with a greasy or lanolin base should be avoided, even though acne lesions do not occur on the scalp. Long-term use of such products can cause "pomade acne," a clustering of blackheads on the forehead and temples.

One of the prime temptations with acne is to squeeze and pick at blackheads and plump pimples. Don't. Handling acne blemishes can lead to secondary infections, rupture of follicle walls, and eventually scars. (The extent of scarring in acne, however, is not directly related to the severity of the case. The scarring potential of the skin is the key factor.) Although there are dermatologists who approve of the home use of a blackhead extractor, we advise against it because of the possibility of skin damage.

Since products containing iodides or bromides sometimes exacerbate existing acne or produce eruptions that look like acne, patients are warned against them during acne treatment. Certain drugs, such as cough medicines, sedatives, cold preparations, and multivitamin/mineral combinations, may contain iodides. Some experts advise that since iodides also occur in iodized salt, saltwater fish, shellfish, spinach, cabbage, lettuce, and artichokes, these foods should be avoided during acne treatment.

Most authorities agree that any other type of dietary manipulation usually makes no difference in the severity of acne. With some people, however, it may seem that specific foods do aggravate the disease. The foods commonly suspected are sugar, nuts, chocolate, and fried foods. If any food seems to worsen the acne, try dropping that food from your diet and observe the effect (or lack of one). After a few weeks, reintroduce the food and again note the result. If the experiment convinces you that the food is culpable, try to avoid it. More likely you will find that changes in your diet make no difference and you can eat pretty much what you like.

If careful trial of OTC medications (see pages 152–53) does not help, consult a physician. But know that control of acne may not come with the first round of professional treatment, either. It may help if you keep in mind that acne, which responds slowly to a physician's care, is likely to be even more stubborn with hit-or-miss self-medication. Take heart and have patience; in most cases, improvement can be achieved.

16

Moisturizers

THE YOUTH AND BEAUTY HUSTLE

If all you wanted to do was moisturize your skin, axle grease would probably work quite well. But you doubtless want something a bit more refined—something that will feel, look, and smell pleasant, that will neither irritate your skin nor stain your clothes.

From such a simple need, a mighty industry has grown. Heavy consumer demand, mostly by women, supports hundreds of all-purpose moisturizers on the market, and additional hundreds of face creams that promise to "nourish," "firm," or "tone" as well as moisturize.

Ads in magazines and on TV endlessly promote the products—especially the high-priced ones marketed just for the face. Beautiful women in lustrous makeup smile seductively, selling not just a facial "creme" but youth and dreams. Sometimes the ads are sexy and vague, sometimes they're clinical and detailed.

Compared with the claims for face creams, the claims made for all-purpose moisturizers are usually more modest. Most simply say they'll "soften," "replenish," and "protect" the skin from dryness. A few promise more. One says it "helps heal severe cases of dry skin"; another says that it "ends dry skin" outright. A number contain ingredients that hint at wondrous powers: "special natural protein complex," vitamin E, "cell extracts," aloe, collagen, elastin.

Women may not be taken in by the more fanciful claims and ingredients in all-purpose moisturizers. When CU surveyed women readers of *Consumer Reports* in 1986, we found that most repondents had realistic expectations of an all-purpose moisturizing lotion. They didn't expect it to cure dry skin, just to soothe it and make it feel softer.

Sales of moisturizers and face creams have rocketed in recent years, for several reasons. For one, the number and type of products have proliferated, as manufacturers have taken a divide-and-conquer approach:

They divide the human anatomy into regions, then market a skin-care product for each region. (That strategy seems to be working; most of the women readers we surveyed said they used a separate, and more expensive, product on their face.)

Does a skin-care product for the face that costs ten times as much as another work any better? No. In fact, in a 1986 home-use test of 48 products by 600 women, we found that quite the opposite was true. We paid from as little as 10 cents per ounce for some store brands to as much as $6.10 per ounce—an astonishingly wide range considering that all the products are so similar in the way they work. If anything, price tended to be a *reverse* indicator of quality.

WHAT A MOISTURIZER CAN AND CAN'T DO

The skin is composed of many layers. The very top layer, called the stratum corneum, or horny layer, is composed of dead cells. Nothing much larger than simple chemical molecules can penetrate that layer. If that layer is to remain supple and flexible, it must be kept moist.

Living cells from deeper layers in the skin supply moisture to the stratum corneum, which, in turn, surrenders moisture to the outside air through evaporation. In normal skin, the rate of water loss is low enough to keep the stratum corneum's water content reasonably high. If, however, the outer layer loses water more rapidly than the cells below can replenish it, the stratum corneum dries out and becomes inflexible and brittle.

The only way that you can alleviate dry skin is to restore the proper balance of moisture to the stratum corneum. Moisturizers can help do this in two ways.

First, most moisturizers contain some kind of oil, which helps retard the evaporation of water. Normally your skin produces enough oil on its own to form an adequate barrier. But various factors such as harsh environments or soaps and detergents can strip the skin of its natural oils. Some people don't have much oil to begin with, having inherited a tendency toward dry skin. And for most people, oil production slows with age.

Moisturizers also work through humectants—ingredients that attract and hold water as it passes to the skin surface through the stratum corneum. Humectants (glycerin is one) can also attract water from the air, but that trick works best in humid environments—where you need a moisturizer least. Humectants also help keep the preparations from drying out while still in the bottle.

Because the main objective of moisturizing is to keep water in contact with the skin, the best time to apply a moisturizer is after you bathe and pat dry, while your skin is still slightly damp.

A moisturizer works only on the surface of the skin—smoothing, softening, and plumping up dead cells—and its effects are only temporary. No matter how expensive a moisturizer is, and no matter what special ingredients it contains, it won't "penetrate deeply" into the layers of the skin, "nourish" the skin, or cure dry skin.

Ad claims made for moisturizers are somewhat limited by the regulations of the U.S. Food and Drug Administration (FDA), which say that any product claiming to affect the body's function or structure is a drug, not a cosmetic. The classification makes a big difference: Drugs have to be approved by the FDA before they can be sold to the public; manufacturers must first prove the products are safe and serve their intended purpose.

Some of the claims made recently for so-called anti-aging creams (with names like *Anti-Age Daytime Skin Treatment, Future Perfect Micro-Targeted SkinGel,* and *Millennium*) would seem to classify them as drugs, not cosmetics. Manufacturers initially claimed these products eliminated wrinkles by helping to "rebuild the intercellular network of your skin," by working "on and within the epidermis to accelerate the natural cell renewal process," or by otherwise altering the skin structure. In 1988, after deliberating for a year, the FDA warned cosmetic firms that their merchandise would be seized unless such claims were dropped. For the time being, at least, the marketing propaganda seems to have become somewhat more restrained.

Retin-A: Youth Cream?

Retin-A is another story. When a study appeared in the *Journal of the American Medical Association* in 1988, the media focused its attention on what many hoped would be a true "youth cream," a "face-lift in a tube."

The prescription acne remedy tretinoin (see page 154), trade name Retin-A, appeared also to be capable of reversing the skin's aging response to sun exposure. Mild improvement had been observed in 30 patients who completed the study. However, the benefits have not been shown to be permanent. And there are side effects—including skin irritation, increased susceptibility to sunburn, and, in some patients, severe dermatitis. (Ten patients dropped out before the end of the trial, including three with severe dermatitis.)

As of this writing, the manufacturer is conducting clinical trials in hopes of obtaining FDA approval to market Retin-A as an antiwrinkle cream. However, widespread prescribing at this time seems premature in view of some doubts about long-term safety.

ENTICING INGREDIENTS AND WHAT THEY DO

Since 1975, the FDA has required that cosmetic labels list all ingredients. That's a help: If you know you're allergic to certain ingredients, you can watch for them. Less helpful is the star billing on the front of the label for certain enticing ingredients, such as the following.

Collagen and Elastin   Collagen is a protein substance found in connective tissue, cartilage, and bone. The dermis, which forms up to 85 percent of the thickness of skin, consists mainly of interlaced collagen fibers. Elastin, which is responsible for making the skin supple and flexible, consists of springlike fibers that run between the collagen fibers. When you're young, collagen and elastin fibers form a tight-knit network. But as you age, those fibers tend to deteriorate. The dermis loses its support and begins to bunch and fold underneath the epidermis. But the epidermis retains its original size, and so those folds appear as wrinkles.

Unfortunately, you can't send your skin reinforcements by smearing on a cream that contains new collagen fibers, though some manufacturers might like you to think so. Collagen and elastin molecules are just too big to penetrate the stratum corneum and work their way down to the dermal layer.

That's not to say these ingredients don't do anything for you. Both collagen and elastin are good at binding moisture to the stratum corneum, especially at low humidities. And they give moisturizing creams and lotions a satiny feel.

Lanolin and Petrolatum Lanolin is wool fat secreted from the oil glands of sheep. Petrolatum is just another name for petroleum jelly. Both retard evaporation of water from the stratum corneum by setting up a barrier on the skin. Pure lanolin can cause mild allergic reactions in some people. But used as a component in a moisturizer, it smooths and softens the skin. Lanolin also makes a cream more spreadable and helps it adhere better to the skin. Petroleum jelly has long been a favorite to apply to a baby's bottom because it's gentle and it forms a barrier to protect the skin from irritation. Plain old petroleum jelly works as a moisturizer for adults, too. But it's greasy, and it tends to rub off on clothes.

Cocoa Butter This solid fat is from the roasted seeds of the cacao tree; the seeds are also the source of cocoa and chocolate. Cocoa butter is a useful ingredient in cosmetic products because it melts at room temperature. Like other oils, cocoa butter works by slowing the evaporation of moisture from the stratum corneum.

Aloe An extract from the succulent plant *Aloe vera,* aloe is a soothing and mild humectant. It can't heal, nourish, or rejuvenate the skin, however.

Vitamin E Vitamin E has been touted for years as having special properties for the skin. One medical consultant described it as "a large, slimy molecule that works like other oils to set up a barrier to evaporation." The problem with vitamin E is that it is a potential allergen and can cause very itchy skin rashes.

In choosing a moisturizer, try to ignore those seductive ads for expensive products. Remember that 600 CU panelists who didn't know the price thought the cheaper, plainer lotions did the best job.

17

Dandruff and Shampoos

Dandruff is a scalp problem, not a hair problem, and for most people it's less of a problem than advertisements would have you believe.

Oiliness and flakiness of the scalp are normal. The human scalp, even at its healthiest, shows a mild degree of scaling; the skin all over the body continually sloughs off bits of its dead outer layer. On the scalp, sebaceous glands add their oily secretion (sebum) to the dead skin scales, forming dandruff.

Back in the days when people washed their hair only once every week or two, this sign of the normal replenishment of scalp skin could easily drop from the hair and turn into an ugly social problem. But people now typically wash their hair almost every day, often enough to wash away the flakes before they fall. In fact, there's nothing wrong with washing your hair as often as you want. Most people, consequently, have no need for a special dandruff shampoo.

HOW SHAMPOOS WORK

The primary function of ordinary shampoo is to remove dirt, dead skin scales, and excess sebum from the hair. The ingredients that do the work are long molecules called surfactants. One end of these molecules is attracted to oil, the other to water. That allows them to grab sebum and whatever dirt it contains and rinse it out of your hair.

Soap, once the main cleaning ingredient in shampoos, is one type of surfactant. But soap reacts with the minerals in hard water, leaving a scummy film on hair. Such a film can be removed with an acidic rinse; that's why people rinsed their hair with lemon juice or vinegar or even beer, which is mildly acidic.

Shampoo manufacturers have since turned to surfactants less trouble-some than soaps. These ingredients are often called detergents, to differentiate them from soaps. Many are derived from the fatty acids of coconuts—hence "essential fatty acids" and "coco-" ingredients.

There are dozens of these surfactants, each with its own properties. Some are much milder than the name *detergent* implies—they might remove dirt but little sebum, or they might not sting if they get into your eyes. Others are especially effective at penetrating and removing oil. Some clean but don't foam; others produce a rich lather. Some leave hair looking better than others do. A manufacturer usually uses several surfactants in a shampoo, one being the principal cleaning agent and the others there to modify its effect. The range of surfactants and their possible combinations provide lots of room for claims of "special" formulations.

Alkaline substances such as detergents tend to leave the hair fluffy; acidic substances such as cream rinses or lemon juice (or beer) tend to smooth it down. That's the origin of the fuss some companies make over their "pH balanced" formulas. Yet the fluffing effect of detergents used in shampoos quickly fades. And most shampoos these days are formulated to be, if not acidic, at least not very alkaline. That's typically done by adding citric acid.

Don't let yourself be intimidated into thinking you must spend a lot of money on a "hair care system" in order to have clean, "healthy" hair. As far as we can tell, relatively inexpensive shampoos contain perfectly adequate cleaning and conditioning ingredients. If you want to spend money on an expensive shampoo, do it knowing that you're indulging your psyche, not your hair.

DANDRUFF SHAMPOOS

While most people don't need a medicated shampoo, some may choose to try one if frequent washing with an ordinary shampoo doesn't control the flaking. These antidandruff formulas are a special subclass of shampoo, considered by the U.S. Food and Drug Administration (FDA) to be—and therefore regulated as—drugs rather cosmetics.

The precise cause of excessive scalp flaking is unknown. Sometimes the production of oily secretions and dead skin scales speeds up until the flaking is definitely excessive. But the transition from the normal to the abnormal state can be so gradual that it is difficult to tell when one condition ends and the other begins. There is no basis for assuming, as some advertisers do, that germs are the primary cause of dandruff, and that an antiseptic shampoo is the cure. Indeed, although severe dandruff can be controlled, it cannot be cured. Spontaneous periods of improvement are common, a fact that casts doubt on all testimonials for cures with any particular product.

The FDA has judged five ingredients used in over-the-counter (OTC) dandruff shampoos to be safe and effective: coal-tar preparations (such as *Denorex* and *Tegrin*), salicylic acid *(P&S, X-Seb),* selenium sulfide *(Selsun),* zinc pyrithione *(Head & Shoulders, Sebulin, Zincon),* and sulfur preparations, which usually also contain salicylic acid *(Sebulex, Vanseb).*

Severe flaking can be a symptom of certain diseases, notably seborrheic dermatitis and psoriasis. Such conditions require diagnosis by a physician, who may prescribe special treatment beyond those OTC preparations.

There is no evidence that changes in diet or the addition of vitamins or minerals can control the development of dandruff or affect the quality of the hair in the slightest way. Nor is there any evidence that exposure of the scalp or head to sunlight either prevents or cures any type of scalp disorder.

Many men worry that dandruff might lead to baldness. Although severe dandruff and "male pattern" baldness (beginning at the temples and progressing to form a "widow's peak") may occur simultaneously, no cause-and-effect relationship between them has ever been shown. Dandruff and scalp oiliness can last for years without leading to the slightest thinning of the hair.

Most people who buy medicated shampoos fear being ostracized by a dandruff-phobic society—spurred on by advertisers for antidandruff products. These social consequences may be reason enough. But the fact is that the medical consequences of dandruff are few, if any. Some dermatologists maintain that dandruff requires treatment. But there is little evidence that scalp itching—the main symptom of dandruff other than "unsightly" white flakes—responds better to medicated shampoos than to ordinary ones.

18

Baldness: Is There Hope?

HAIR REGROWTH AND MINOXIDIL

Surefire cures for baldness have been around ever since man learned to talk fast. But lately there's a dramatic new twist to the promise: a remedy with medical credentials and FDA approval. The source of excitement is a drug called minoxidil, which is mixed in an alcohol-based solution and rubbed on the scalp. Unlike the snake oils of the past, minoxidil has been tested in controlled studies. And while it didn't always halt baldness or regrow hair, it did work on some men to some degree.

Minoxidil was originally approved by the U.S. Food and Drug Administration (FDA) in 1979 as a treatment for hypertension, to be marketed as Loniten tablets by Upjohn Co. While waiting for FDA approval to market minoxidil as a baldness treatment as well, Upjohn began selling the drug for that purpose in some 40 other countries, including Canada and most of Europe. In 1988, the FDA approved a 2 percent topical solution of minoxidil, to be marketed for baldness under the brand name Rogaine.

Many doctors across the United States hadn't waited for the FDA to act. After all, there is no federal law that prevents physicians from prescribing any approved drug for whatever use they see fit—although it is illegal for a drug manufacturer to *market* a drug for uses other than those approved. A 1985 survey conducted among U.S. dermatologists found that 72 percent were already prescribing minoxidil for hair loss. Such wide acceptance by dermatologists suggested a vote of confidence—a confidence no doubt inspired by the outcome of an Upjohn-sponsored minoxidil trial.

The trial involved some 2300 participants treated at 27 different medical centers. Among those using a 2 percent minoxidil solution for one year, 8 percent were described as experiencing dense new hair growth and 31 percent moderate new hair growth. The remaining 61 percent showed little or no new hair growth.

A success rate of 39 percent many seem modest. But compared with the zero success rate for all other baldness remedies tried before, the results were stunning. Many bald or balding men would jump at a 4-in-10 chance of growing hair.

A close look at the minoxidil studies, however, indicates that those widely publicized odds may be overstated.

The Discovery of Minoxidil

The discovery of minoxidil's hair-growing properties came entirely by accident. When Loniten tablets were prescribed for high blood pressure, 80 percent of the users experienced hair growth on some part of the body, often on the forehead or the upper cheek. It didn't take long for researchers to wonder what would happen if they compounded minoxidil into a topical solution and had balding men rub it into their scalps.

But the researchers also had to worry about its safety. When taken for hypertension, minoxidil tablets can have serious side effects—so much so that the drug is not recommended for use until safer antihypertension drugs have been tried first. Adverse effects can include a rapid heart rate, fainting, vomiting, difficulty breathing, and accumulation of fluid around the heart. So even though topical minoxidil would be used for a cosmetic purpose, it had to be tested for safety and efficacy before it could be marketed.

In 1983, Upjohn initiated its trial of minoxidil as a baldness remedy. Nearly all of the 2300 subjects were men, aged 18 to 49, with male-pattern baldness. All were in good health, with no hypertension or heart problems that might make the side effects of minoxidil more dangerous.

Male-pattern baldness is by far the most common form of hair loss, eventually affecting two out of three men. Such baldness is inherited from either side of the family. (It's not caused by poor circulation in the scalp, vitamin deficiencies, or any of the other factors you might read about in ads for products claiming to retard hair loss.) Some hair follicles have a genetic predisposition to bind with certain male hormones, which act to shut the follicles down. Hair follicles at the temples and on the crown of the head are more susceptible than those on the sides and back. Women also experience hair loss as they age, but it's more often manifested by thinning hair all over the head.

Each of the participants in the 1983 study applied minoxidil to the scalp twice a day for a year. But even after four months, one conclusion became apparent: Minoxidil was growing some hair on some men.

Just why minoxidil worked was a matter of conjecture. The drug dilates the smaller blood vessels, which in turn lowers blood pressure. But dilation of blood vessels in the scalp isn't what grows the hair; no other similarly acting drug has demonstrated the same hair-restoration effect as minoxidil. "The most plausible theory is that minoxidil somehow stimulates the matrix cell of the hair follicle to regrow when it was destined to turn off," said Richard De Villez, M.D., Upjohn's director of dermatology, in 1988. "It's an overcoming of the genetic propensity to shut down. But we don't know how minoxidil modifies the metabolic activity of that cell."

How Effective Is Minoxidil

What percentage of men actually get new hair—and how much—still isn't clear. The oft-quoted 4-in-10 chance appears unduly optimistic.

The study participants were selected to favor those who were likely to do best on minoxidil. Younger men do much better than older ones, and the study excluded men over 49. Similarly, minoxidil works best on those with small areas of baldness. The study excluded men who were very bald—those with hair only on the sides and a smooth, shiny crown. Finally, minoxidil rarely works for a receding hairline. (For reasons that aren't understood, it can restore hair on the top of the head but not at the temples.) The study excluded men who were growing bald only at the temples.

By confining the participants to men who were relatively young, not completely bald, and not bald just at the temples, the Upjohn study guaranteed a better result than would have been the case if men with all types of baldness had been enrolled at random.

Another weakness of the study was the short-lived role of the control group. In a medical study, it's important to have a control group taking a placebo, a substance having no pharmacological effect.

The Upjohn study used a control group for only four months of the year-long trial. After four months, the placebo group was switched over to minoxidil. By then, Upjohn reasoned, many participants in either group who weren't growing new hair would assume they were in the control group, lose interest, and drop out, thus compromising the eventual results.

Interestingly enough, however, the results after four months indicated that some members of the placebo group seemed to be growing new hair. According to assessments by doctors supervising the studies, 32 percent of the patients using minoxidil had new "non-vellus" hair growth after four months—but so did 20 percent of the placebo group. (Vellus hairs are the tiny, colorless "peach fuzz," which the doctors ignored.)

What was happening? Could the act of rubbing the scalp, or the contents of the placebo, be having an effect? Many dermatologists strongly doubt it. (The placebo consisted of the minoxidil solution minus minoxidil: alcohol, water, and a solvent called propylene glycol.) The most likely answer, they say, was that the optimism of the doctors supervising the studies unconsciously biased their appraisal of hair growth.

"I can think of no likely explanation of why the placebo group did well other than observer bias," said Robert Stern, M.D., associate professor of dermatology at Harvard Medical School and head of the FDA expert advisory panel that studied the data on topical minoxidil. Counting hairs "is an extraordinarily tedious and error-prone process," Stern told CU. "It's not so objective that biases don't enter into it."

To what extent did such bias inflate the one-year appraisal of minoxidil's success rate? Without a valid control group for comparison, no one can say. "I don't think anyone can really tell you what happened at 12 months because of the lack of a placebo," said Stern. "Those are the facts of doing unblinded studies with an agent people think will work."

Another key question is how much new hair is actually sprouting. It turns out that the assessment of new hair growth in the study applied only to what happened in a one-inch circle on the crown of the head, not the entire scalp. And the crown is the area where minoxidil is most effective. So even the 8 percent in the "dense" regrowth category weren't necessarily getting back a full head of hair.

Moreover, the categories "dense" and "moderate" didn't actually represent a specified number of new hairs grown back. They were instead the subjective assessments of the physicians running the studies at the 27 centers. Upjohn's De Villez said that in his view "moderate" would be defined as "a significant coverage that would cover over 50 percent of the balding area." But in a 1987 article published in the British medical journal *The Lancet,* three European dermatologists evaluating the Upjohn studies reported a very different impression. They concluded that "a more graphic description of 'moderate' growth might be 'mostly fluff.'"

CU asked several of the U.S. dermatologists who studied minoxidil what their appraisal was. Their responses were often significantly less enthusiastic than the rosy picture that emerged from press accounts. "I think at best one-third of the 'moderate' group had a good change in hair patterns," said Larry Millikan, M.D., chairman of dermatology at Tulane University Medical Center. "Many of the 'moderates' get increased vellus hairs, which decreases the shine some but doesn't give significant change." Referring to a standardized scale depicting 12 relative degrees of baldness, Millikan said of his minoxidil patients: "Basically we didn't have anyone who moved up more than one on the scale. No one got a full head of hair. No one grew hair at the temples."

Stern said that, from his review of the pertinent literature, he didn't believe the efficacy of minoxidil approached the 39 percent total that the Upjohn data suggest. "In well-selected individuals, with hair loss at the crown of the head, with vellus hairs present in fair density, my best estimate is that about one-fifth of the people are helped in terms of increasing hairs."

The authors of the *Lancet* article were less optimistic. They concluded that for "90 percent or so" of men with hair loss, minoxidil "does nothing."

Two important questions about minoxidil's efficacy weren't addressed by the Upjohn studies. First, what happens after one year—even if you keep using the drug twice a day? Do you keep the new hair growth, do you grow more, or do you regress? Second, does minoxidil have any effect in slowing or stopping hair loss?

Although many minoxidil studies have been published in medical journals, as of this writing only two have followed participants beyond one year. They dealt mainly with patients who had shown new hair growth the first year, since most of the others lost interest and dropped out. Both studies indicated that there was some regression despite continued minoxidil use. Many of the participants, it turned out, were losing some hair they had grown during that first year.

One study was conducted by Judith Koperski, M.D., a dermatologist at the Scripps Clinic and Research Foundation in La Jolla, California. She followed 33 patients for 30 months, making periodic counts of hairs in the one-inch circle at the crown. Men who aren't balding have roughly 1000 hairs in that one-inch circle. The mean hair count of the balding patients at the start of the study was 119. It peaked after one year at 353. After 30 months, however, it had fallen to 250.

Another negative development also surfaced with time. At 21 months, the diameter of the area that was balding had "decreased significantly," Koperski reported. But by 30 months, she noted, the trend had reversed. Even though most of the participants had more hair on top than when they started, the diameter of the bald area was not significantly different from the initial diameter.

In the second study, conducted by Elise A. Olsen, M.D., a dermatologist at Duke University Medical School, 21 men were evaluated for a period extending from one year through 33 months on minoxidil treatment. On average, their mean hair count in the one-inch circle rose slightly during the period, but there was also an unpleasant surprise. At the end of one year, Olsen had rated 15 of the men as having at least moderate regrowth of hair overall. But after 33 months, that appraisal applied to only one man in the group.

Why the startling drop-off, especially since the group overall wasn't losing hair from the one-inch circle on top? Olsen said that some men lost hair in other areas. And while a majority of the group did gain a bit more hair in the one-inch circle, nine men regressed in that area.

The two studies raise the possibility that minoxidil might not be successful over the long run in preserving whatever gains occur the first year. Meanwhile, minoxidil has to be used indefinitely for any chance of retaining new hair. And there can be no skimping. One study demonstrated a significant difference in retaining the hair when minoxidil is applied twice a day, as recommended, rather than just once a day.

Whatever the shortcomings of minoxidil in growing and keeping new hair, a drug that blocked future hair loss would still find a ready and enthusiastic market. Men with a family history of baldness might want to start using it at the first sign of hair loss.

None of the minoxidil studies published as of this writing has explored this issue, however. Such a study is difficult to carry out because everyone loses hair at a different rate.

De Villez at Upjohn said in 1988 that there are "anecdotal reports" that hair loss stabilizes with minoxidil. "My feeling, and that of most investigators, is that the first thing the patients tell you is they noticed they were no longer shedding hair like they had before. But it's too tenuous to make a claim."

How Safe Is Minoxidil?

Although minoxidil can be a troublesome drug when taken orally for hypertension, rubbing it on the scalp appears to be safe for most men. After one year of daily use, the 2300 participants in the 1983 Upjohn trials showed no serious side effects.

One major finding was that relatively little of the drug was penetrating the scalp and entering the bloodstream. In safety data submitted to the FDA, Upjohn reported that concentrations of minoxidil in the blood of the subjects ranged from 1 to 10 percent of those blood levels commonly seen in patients taking the drug orally.

The most common side effect was itching of the scalp, which occurred in 3 percent of the participants. In some cases, itching may be caused by the solution itself (alcohol can dry the skin); in others, it may indicate an allergic reaction to the drug. Upjohn recommends that users who experience itching stop applying minoxidil for a few days and start again when the itching subsides. If it recurs, then a physician should be consulted to check the possibility of an allergic reaction.

There also were scattered reports of chest pains, blood-pressure or pulse-rate changes, shortness of breath, and fluid retention, but their occurrence was no greater in the minoxidil group than in the placebo group. Some experts feel, however, that a short-term study among healthy men isn't conclusive enough to rule out the possibility of such effects from minoxidil, and they advise periodic checkups for those using the drug, particularly in the early months.

One small study conducted in Canada found significant increases in heart rate and cardiac output (the volume of blood the heart pumps) in men on topical minoxidil. No such findings were noted in any of the U.S. studies, however, and many researchers are skeptical of that report.

While the Upjohn studies are reassuring, all of the participants were healthy and relatively young. Topical minoxidil hasn't yet been tested in men with cardiovascular problems, and many physicians suspect it might be hazardous for that group. Since cardiovascular problems increase with age, some experts caution that any risk of side effects from minoxidil is likely to be higher in men 50 and over than in a younger group.

The lack of serious side effects among the study participants doesn't mean minoxidil is safe for everyone. If you're using minoxidil or intend to try it, be sure to consult your personal physician about the advisability of periodic checkups, particularly if you're age 50 or older.

What Price Fuzz?

Upjohn's minoxidil product, Rogaine, comes in a bottle containing a one-month supply, with a choice of rub-on or spray applicators. The applicators are designed so that you get just the right dosage, one milliliter per application. You apply it not only to balding spots but also to adjacent areas that might go bald. (It must be used only on dry hair and scalp, and you have to avoid getting it wet for at least an hour afterward.) The price of a one-month supply ranges widely, starting at $50.

Then there's the cost of doctor visits, to determine if you're a suitable candidate and to monitor your progress if you are. Medical insurance is unlikely to cover any of these expenses, because topical minoxidil is used for cosmetic reasons. Thus, it could cost you anywhere from several hundred dollars to well over $1000 just to find out if you are among the small percentage of men who might grow some hair on the crown by rubbing minoxidil into the scalp twice a day for a year.

Nor do costs end if and when hair comes in. The studies so far indicate that most of the hair growth appears between eight months and one year after beginning treatment. But to try to maintain that hair, you have to apply the drug twice a day for the rest of your life. If you stop using it, all the new hair will fall out within three or four months.

No one on minoxidil is going to start off entirely bald and end up with a thick head of hair. At best, you can hope that a partially bald area on top of your head gets filled in to some extent.

The odds of conjuring some hair out of the minoxidil bottle can depend on several factors. Are you under 30? Have you been losing hair for less than five years? Is the hair loss mostly on the crown of the head instead of in a receding hairline? Is the bald spot on top relatively small in diameter? Are there still some hairs left on that bald spot? Although there's no way of predicting with certainty which individuals will respond favorably, the more "yes" answers to these questions, the better your odds.

Some dermatologists think minoxidil is more significant as a medical stepping-stone than it is as a treatment for baldness. The first substance actually proven to grow hair in *any* amount, minoxidil does offer some encouragement for future research. In the meantime, though, you pay your money and you take your chance—most likely a slim one.

HAIR TRANSPLANTS: THE SURGICAL ALTERNATIVE

If you have time, money, and a stoic attitude toward pain, hair-transplant surgery can be a way of fighting hair loss. It involves a series of operations that extract plugs of scalp from the sides and back of your head, where hair grows densely, and implant them on top and in front, where you're going bald. Hair transplanted from the back or side of the head will continue to grow as it would have at its original site. A skilled surgeon can take hair from the fringes of your scalp without making that area look sparse.

The procedure, which usually isn't covered by medical insurance, can cost as much as $15,000 and takes a year or two to complete. Despite the time and expense, an estimated 250,000 American men each year elect to have the surgery.

Hair-transplant surgery requires a series of visits for treatment. The doctor begins by injecting a local anesthetic into the areas where the surgery will take place. Then a circular punch that looks like a small cookie cutter is used to remove tiny pieces of scalp, each containing about 8 to 15 hair follicles. They're placed in spots on the bald scalp that have been cut with a similar instrument. The donor sites are closed with stitches, while the area that received the transplant is bandaged for a day or so. The grafts have to be spaced far enough apart to ensure adequate nourishment from surrounding blood vessels. That's why hair transplants are done in stages, often with about 30 grafts at a time, then at least a three-week wait.

The surgeon may also perform a procedure called scalp reduction, which decreases the area of bald scalp that the transplants have to fill. A strip of skin is cut out of the bald area and the edges of the scalp are sewn together, which moves the hair on the sides of the head closer to the top. A scalp-reduction procedure may cost $1500 to $2000.

If everything goes well, side effects from the surgery should be relatively minor. There's overnight pain, temporary swelling that might appear after a day or two, and a sensation of numbness that could last for weeks or months until nerve endings regrow. Extraction of the scalp plugs leaves faint scars, but if the procedure is done correctly, the scars should be hidden by the remaining hair. More serious but rarer side effects include postoperative bleeding, which may require additional stitches, and infection, which is treated with antibiotics.

There can also be a psychological burden. If the bald area is large, the healing and hair-growing process may be visible to the world. (Senator William Proxmire, one of the most famous hair-transplant patients, found his progress monitored by photographers and TV cameras.)

There's considerable debate among dermatologists about whether hair transplants offer enough cosmetic improvement to be worth the time, cost, and discomfort. A major problem is finding a surgeon who can produce good results. Since any licensed physician in the United States can perform the surgery, it's easy to end up with transplanted tufts of hair that look like uneven rows of corn. You could also find yourself with a surgeon who uses controversial techniques. One such procedure is to transplant a large flap of scalp instead of tiny grafts. Not only does that increase the chance of visible scarring, but in some cases the flaps won't take, and you lose all the transplanted hair.

When seeking a surgeon, ignore advertisements by big assembly-line hair clinics. Instead, consult a dermatologist whose practice does *not* include hair transplant surgery. You can ask your own doctor for a referral or call the dermatology department of a local medical school. The dermatologist should be able to give you an objective appraisal of whether you're a good candidate for a hair transplant. If you are, then ask for the name of a qualified surgeon. The surgeon should be willing to show you before-and-after photos of previous patients to give you an idea of what to expect.

IV

TEETH and GUMS

19

Care of Teeth and Gums

Tooth decay and gum disease are two of the most prevalent public-health problems in the United States. They're both largely preventable. Though dentists and hygienists play crucial roles in prevention, the responsibility for good dental health cannot be left only to the professionals. Diligent care at home—through a conscientious oral-hygiene regimen—is essential. Toothpastes, certain mouth rinses, dental floss, and dental sealants can all contribute to that regimen. Fluoride is most important of all.

TOOTH DECAY: THE EARLY PROBLEM

Only the common cold is a more prevalent health problem than tooth decay. Dental cavities, or caries (as the disease process is called), afflict about 90 percent of Americans, who endure the dentist's drill for some 200 million fillings annually.

The good news is that the rate of tooth decay among children has dropped sharply in the past two decades. In 1988, the National Institute of Dental Research, a part of the National Institutes of Health (NIH), reported that nearly 50 percent of the nation's schoolchildren have no tooth decay at all—as opposed to an estimated 28 percent in the early 1970s.

Public-health experts report that the majority—up to 90 percent—of dental caries could be avoided with currently available measures. But many people remain unaware of what the most effective measures are, and some dentists still aren't even offering a full range of preventive services.

PREVENTING TOOTH DECAY: HOW EFFECTIVE IS THE TIME-WORN ADVICE?

In the good old days, the road to bristling dental health was seemingly well marked: Brush and floss daily, restrict between-meal sweets, and visit your dentist every six months. That advice still makes good sense, say the experts, but it's not the most effective way to prevent tooth decay.

Brushing and Flossing These are important for removing dental plaque—a thin, sticky, transparent film that forms continually on tooth surfaces. Certain bacteria, especially those on the inner surface of the plaque, produce acids that can attack the tooth enamel. Plaque can also build up over time and harden into a complex material called dental calculus, or tartar. The mixture of deposits can lead to gum disease and tooth loss.

Logically, then, removing plaque daily should prevent tooth decay. "A clean tooth never decays," says an old dental adage. But the question is, "How clean?" The answer, unfortunately, is cleaner than most children and adults are realistically able to achieve.

School-based studies extending for periods of up to three years have examined the effect of thorough plaque removal once a day on the oral health of children. The controlled studies showed that such a regimen is beneficial for preventing gum inflammation but not significantly effective in reducing cavities. These studies and similar research with adults suggest that an even more frequent plaque-removal regimen would be required to reduce caries appreciably—a commitment unlikely to be kept by most adults, let alone by young children and teenagers.

Restricting Sweets Dietary advice about sugar presents a similar confrontation with reality. There's little doubt among dental experts that tooth decay is promoted by frequent consumption of sweets—confections and baked goods—especially between meals (when the sugar is likely to remain longer in the mouth). Sugars of various kinds serve as nutrients for the bacteria in plaque. But years of urging the public to restrict its intake of sugary foods have not countered the effect of the heavy promotion for such foods, and many dental professionals see scant hope of changing the nation's eating habits in that regard.

Moreover, there are sugars in many processed foods that aren't obviously sweet, and in many fruits as well. While cutting out candy bars and cookies can play a part in reducing the risk of developing caries, it's not practical to eliminate all sugars from the diet just to prevent tooth decay.

Regular Dental Visits   Since the early 1970s, professional interest in preventive measures has increased. But to some extent, routine dental treatment still consists of treating dental problems rather than preventing them.

Despite the limitations of the traditional approaches to caries prevention, most people accord them high priority. In one typical survey of public perceptions about tooth decay, conducted in Minnesota in 1980, 653 adults were asked what they thought was the best way to avoid getting cavities. Sixty-one percent chose oral-hygiene measures; 15 percent said visiting the dentist; and 12 percent advised avoiding sweets. Only about 1 percent mentioned the use of fluoride (beyond its use in toothpastes). Actually, the use of multiple sources of fluoride—in municipal or school water supplies, in supplements (tablets or drops), or in dentifrices, mouth rinses, and other topical applications—has proved by far the most effective approach to preventing tooth decay.

Since trying to alter the nation's oral-hygiene and eating habits has proved unrealistic, public-health officials have for many years focused their efforts on strengthening the nation's teeth. Specifically, public-health strategy has been to increase the resistance of the tooth itself to decay. In addition to wider use of fluoride, a major recent component of the newer approach is the application of dental sealants—thin watertight coatings that protect vulnerable surfaces of the teeth.

FLUORIDE: THE BEST PROTECTION AGAINST TOOTH DECAY

Fluoride protects teeth in a number of ways, some of which are only partially understood.

One of the initial benefits is its effect on developing teeth. Before the teeth erupt from the gums, fluoride ingested from drinking water or from fluoride supplements is readily incorporated into the tooth enamel. This fluoride-rich enamel increases the tooth's resistance to the acid attack generated by plaque bacteria. Until the early 1970s, many dental scientists thought that the increased resistance conferred during tooth development was fluoride's principal or sole effect. This suggested that fluoride's protective benefits were gained mainly or exclusively during childhood. Since that time, however, research has disclosed that fluoride also acts in other important ways to protect teeth.

Fluoride from drinking water, some toothpastes, or other topical applications is now known to mix with saliva and diffuse into the plaque on teeth. This topical fluoride appears to have two major actions, although the complete process has not been fully sorted out. Tooth decay begins when the acid attack on tooth enamel causes mineral loss of calcium and phosphate. One effect of fluoride is to improve "remineralization" of the enamel by increasing the rate of calcium and phosphate uptake and decreasing the solubility of the enamel, helping to counteract that mineral loss. In another important action, fluoride appears to affect the metabolism of the bacteria, impairing their ability to produce acid from sugars. Both of these effects—strengthening the enamel and inhibiting acid production—benefit adults as well as children.

An additional benefit, which may apply strictly to adults, is the effect fluoride is believed to have in inhibiting the development of surface caries on the root. As age or gum disease causes the gum line to recede, exposed root surfaces become more vulnerable to acid attack. Fluoride is believed to protect the root surface, or cementum, in much the same way it does the enamel.

In short, fluoride is a versatile weapon against tooth decay. Lifelong access to fluoridated drinking water imparts the fullest benefits. Fluoridation of community water supplies, says the U.S. Public Health Service, "can reduce the incidence of dental caries by about 65 percent, reduce the need for multiple-surface fillings, crowns, and extractions, and significantly increase the number of children who are completely free of cavities."

Fluoride and Public Policy

Fluoridation is the most economical way to provide fluoride to everyone. The annual cost of treating a municipal water supply averages about 25 cents a person.

Nevertheless, more than 70 million Americans live in communities that have central water systems but don't fluoridate them. The reasons for opposition to fluoridation are complex. Some people are concerned that fluoridation poses a conflict between the public's interest in dental health and the rights of individuals to choose which risks they will assume. Political opponents of fluoridation often exaggerate the risks, claiming it poses hazards that, in fact, are simply not supported by any credible scientific evidence.

Extensive studies carried out over more than 40 years have established conclusively that fluoridation of community water supplies provides major dental-health benefits and that the procedure is acceptably safe. Numerous studies have found no reliable evidence that fluoridation poses a risk to the public health. Under normal circumstances, the only occasional effect is faint, whitish spotting of the teeth, which is generally visible only to an examining dentist. Public health authorities consider this minor cosmetic risk fully acceptable in light of the benefits of fluoridation. In communities without central water systems, or where fluoridation has not been approved, fluoridation of school water supplies can be an effective and relatively economical alternative for children. Other ways for compensating for the lack of fluoridated drinking water include prescribed dietary supplements during tooth development, professional topical fluoride treatment, and school-based fluoride treatment programs—though some of these measures can be considerably less economical. Even with fluoridated drinking water, topical use of some fluoride toothpastes and mouth rinses can offer added protection.

Cautions About Fluoride

With multiple sources of fluoride available, some caution is necessary to avoid too much of a good thing, especially with young children. While small amounts of fluoride benefit the teeth, prolonged excessive intake can cause undesirable results, ranging from a slight discoloration of the enamel to more serious effects on teeth or bones.

The American Dental Association, for example, advises against giving dietary fluoride supplements to children in communities with fluoridated drinking water or with water supplies that have a natural fluoride content of 0.7 parts per million or higher. Dental experts also recommend that very young children in such communities or those receiving fluoride supplements be taught to limit their use of fluoride dentifrices, since the children may tend to swallow some toothpaste. Once-a-day brushing with a pea-sized quantity or a thin layer of fluoride toothpaste can give adequate protection against tooth decay in such instances. In addition, children under six years old should not use fluoride mouth rinses because they have difficulty rinsing and tend to swallow too much of the liquid.

An important precaution should be followed by kidney patients on dialysis. Since such patients are typically exposed to about 50 to 100 times the amount of fluid consumed by the average person, experts recommend that fluoride—as well as calcium, magnesium, copper, and other trace elements—be removed from tap water before it is used in an artificial kidney machine.

Fluoride does have its limitations. While it reduces the incidence of all types of cavities, it is most effective in preventing those that occur on smooth surfaces, such as the sides of a tooth. It's less effective against cavities that develop on surfaces with pits and fissures, such as the chewing surfaces of the back teeth (molars and premolars). Those surfaces are especially vulnerable to decay because bacteria and food debris can lodge in the tiny pits and fissures.

Over the years, as decay on the smooth surfaces between teeth has approached eradication (in children, at least) tooth decay has increasingly become a pit-and-fissure disease. Fortunately, there's an effective remedy against this type of decay. But it has only recently begun to gain wider acceptance.

SEALING OUT TOOTH DECAY

In 1983, the National Institutes of Health convened a panel of experts in dentistry and public health to evaluate the effectiveness, safety, and use of dental sealants. Ordinarily, such NIH "consensus development conferences" are held to thrash out some reasonable approach to a controversial health issue or practice. In this instance, however, the panel's deliberations and findings were marked by virtual unanimity: Dental sealants, the panel concluded, are a highly effective and safe means of preventing pit-and-fissure caries in children. "Expanding the use of sealants," said the panel, "would substantially reduce the occurrence of dental caries."

Although most people have only recently begun to hear of sealants, these thin, plastic coatings are neither new nor exotic. They were among the first applications of the acid-etching technique now popularly known as "bonding," and some dentists have been placing them on children's teeth for years. What *is* new is the growing recognition among dentists of the value of sealants. Earlier doubts have been largely dispelled. With improvements in the materials and in application techniques, the sealants work well and offer definite advantages for the patient.

Application of sealants is essentially a painless procedure, requiring no anesthetic or drilling. The chewing surfaces of molars and premolars are the areas commonly sealed, and several teeth may be treated at the same time. The surface is first cleaned thoroughly and then etched with a mild acid solution, which removes an extremely thin layer of enamel and makes the surface more porous and retentive. The sealant is then painted on with a small brush in much the same way that nail polish is applied. Some coatings are formulated to "self-cure," or harden by themselves. Others are cured by exposure to a small beam of visible or ultraviolet light from a hand-operated instrument. In either case, the coatings harden rapidly; the entire procedure takes only about 10 minutes or so.

Once the coating hardens, it effectively seals the enamel from any contact with plaque acids. As long as the sealant remains intact, it completely protects the surface against caries. Clinical studies report that most sealants are retained for several years or longer. Indeed, there are now data on good retention after 10 years. If all or part of the sealant is lost, the tooth can be resealed. Even if a sealant is only partially retained, however, it will still provide some protection.

The prime candidates for sealants are children and, to a lesser extent, teenagers. The teeth commonly recommended for sealant application include the molars of the primary teeth and the newly erupted permanent molars and premolars. Fees for sealants vary widely. In private practice, charges may range anywhere from $10 to more than $35 per tooth.

When sealants were first introduced, they were considered experimental, and most dentists—and dental insurers—kept their distance. In recent years, however, advances in application technique, the emergence of accepted guidelines, and the proven efficacy of sealants have eased earlier concerns about their use. Sealants are now increasingly popular and readily available. There are certainly no longer any valid reasons for delaying their use. Bear in mind, however, that sealants are a supplement to—not a substitute for—fluoride and the other oral hygiene strategies (diligent brushing, flossing, and professional cleanings).

GUM DISEASE AND PLAQUE

As plaque advances, it initiates periodontal disease, or pyorrhea—more commonly known as gum disease. The film of plaque extends beneath the gum line into the crevices between the gum and the teeth. Gum disease begins when bacteria form and release toxic substances that irritate and damage adjacent gum tissue. This tissue provides support for the teeth, interlocking with the tooth surface to form part of a complex anchoring system.

In response to the release of bacterial toxins, white blood cells move to the site of the irritation through swollen blood vessels. In addition, antibodies and other products of the immune system migrate to the affected tissue. That results in the redness, swelling, and pain characteristic of gingivitis, the initial and most common form of periodontal disease.

Over a period of time, which can vary from a few years to many years, the inflamed and injured gums pull away from the tooth, forming a pocket that accommodates even more bacteria and their products. As the process continues, the pocket deepens and the infection and inflammation spread to the supporting ligament and bone of the tooth socket. At the same time, the gum tissue may recede or begin to lose its grip on the teeth, which may eventually loosen and fall out. What began as gingivitis has now become periodontitis—the condition mainly responsible for at least some missing teeth in countless Americans and total toothlessness in millions more.

Although teeth are usually not lost to periodontal disease until middle age or later, the damage commonly begins many years earlier. One federal health survey found that 39 percent of children between the ages of 6 and 11 have gingivitis to some degree; for youths between 12 and 17, the percentage was 68 percent. Gingivitis would be rather unimportant were it not the root of periodontitis.

It has been estimated that up to 75 percent of Americans have some degree of periodontal disease, but most of them don't know it. The disease is insidious; typically, it causes damage gradually over many years with few signs of its presence. Obvious symptoms such as pain or loose teeth are not evident until the later stages, when much of the supporting tissue has already been destroyed.

Careful daily brushing and flossing can go a long way toward preventing gum disease. No matter how well you brush and floss, however, some plaque will inevitably survive. Plaque, as mentioned earlier, can harden on the teeth to form a rough scale called dental calculus, or tartar. Calculus occurs both on the crown and along the roots of the teeth. Unless calculus is thoroughly removed, its plaque coating will injure surrounding gum tissue. Calculus itself may also be a repository for bacterial toxins.

Neither brushing nor flossing can remove calculus. That's done by an oral hygienist or a dentist, using special instruments to scrape the calculus and plaque remnants from the teeth. An effective oral-hygiene program must include both daily home care and periodic professional cleaning. Two cleanings per year are generally recommended. But if you don't brush or floss conscientiously—or if you form deposits rapidly—you should probably have more frequent professional cleanings.

No checkup is complete unless your dentist examines your teeth and gums for evidence of periodontal disease. This should consist of more than just a visual inspection. In a thorough evaluation, the dentist will poke around each tooth with a thin instrument—a periodontal probe—to check pocket depth, which indicates the degree of tissue destruction and the severity of periodontitis.

OTHER FACTORS IN GUM DISEASE

Bacterial plaque is the primary cause of periodontal disease, but other factors can affect its onset or course—for good or for ill. Here are the main ones:

Jaw Configuration A bad bite (malocclusion), clenching or grinding the teeth, or abnormal tooth relationships can put a strain on the periodontal ligaments and supporting bone that hold teeth in place. When periodontal inflammation weakens these tissues, the combined stresses increase the risk of tooth loss. In some cases, adjusting the "bite" through orthodontic treatment can help protect such teeth before they're threatened. Increasingly, adults are wearing braces for this reason, as well as for cosmetic benefit.

Restorative Work Fillings or other restorations, such as crowns, should fit flush with the tooth surface. If they overhang at the gum line, it's difficult to keep the gum areas clean and free of plaque, making them more vulnerable to periodontal disease. Faulty restorations can sometimes be filed down; if not, they may need to be replaced.

Tobacco Smoking damages mouth tissues as well as other parts of the body. People who smoke have greater accumulations of plaque and calculus in their mouth and poorer periodontal health. Tobacco chewing is also associated with poor periodontal health, as well as with other oral diseases, including oral cancer.

Medical Conditions Certain conditions can increase susceptibility to periodontal disease: diabetes and some blood disorders—probably because of lowered resistance to infection; pregnancy—probably because of altered hormone levels; and epilepsy—because phenytoin (Dilantin), the drug most often used to control it, causes overgrowth of gum tissue. Good preventive measures—conscientious home care plus regular professional cleanings—are especially important in these situations.

Fluoride As we have discussed, it's long been established that fluoride in all forms dramatically reduces tooth decay. There are some indications that fluoride can also have a beneficial effect on periodontal disease.

Nutrition Though the foods you eat do not play a major role in periodontal disease, it's probably a good idea to moderate your intake of sweets, especially between meals, since sugar encourages the growth of plaque. Some people believe that high doses of vitamin C are good for the gums, but a study of more than 8500 people found no relationship between the level of vitamin-C intake and periodontal disease. Studies in experimental animals, however, indicate that vitamin C may have a subtle effect on tissue resistance to the disease and its progression. The role of other nutrients, such as folic acid, calcium, and phosphorus, is also under investigation.

TREATING GUM DISEASE: TRADITIONAL VERSUS CONTROVERSIAL TECHNIQUES

Your dentist may be able to treat periodontitis with techniques known as "deep scaling" and "root planing." These are similar to the scraping away of calculus done in a routine cleaning, except that finer instruments are inserted farther down the side of the tooth beneath the gum margin—if possible, to the infection at the base of the pocket. A single treatment can sharply reduce bacteria levels in the pocket. In addition, scaling scrapes away the diseased gum tissue adjacent to the tooth. Together with planing the root surface, scaling promotes the growth of healthy gum tissue that can often reattach the tooth.

Scaling has long been used in periodontal therapy, both by itself and in preparation for gum surgery. Studies have shown that deep scaling itself can achieve clinical improvement often equal to surgery. These studies have established deep scaling as the preferred procedure for mild to moderate periodontitis. Even some cases of severe periodontitis—routinely treated surgically in the past—may respond quite well to deep scaling alone, when accompanied by effective personal oral hygiene.

In the 10 to 15 percent of periodontitis cases that do reach the severe stage, dentists in general practice often refer patients to periodontists, who have trained for at least two years beyond dental school to specialize in treating periodontal disease.

People often associate "periodontist" with "periodontal surgery." Surgery, periodontists say, is necessary to eliminate pockets that are too deep or too convoluted for a scaler to reach the infection. Surgery is also called for, they say, when the infection involves the area between the roots of multirooted teeth.

But is such surgery always necessary? Since the late 1970s, a great deal of publicity has accompanied a "conservative, nonsurgical" method for treating periodontal disease. This method has generated a major dental controversy. Dr. Paul Keyes, who worked for 27 years at the National

Institute of Dental Research, developed the technique while treating cases of severe periodontal disease, some of which had not responded to surgery. Since the disease is caused by bacteria, Keyes reasoned, it should be treated like other bacterial infections—with antibacterial agents rather than with surgery.

Thus was born the Keyes technique. Plaque is scraped from beneath the gum line, and the form and movement of the bacteria are examined under a special microscope. If certain types of bacteria are present, the site that contained the plaque is considered diseased. Treatment then focuses on killing the bacteria in a number of ways short of surgery.

Like other dentists and periodontists, Keyes uses deep scaling. But he also attacks the bacteria through a home-care regimen in which the patient applies common antibacterial agents—hydrogen peroxide, baking soda, and salt solutions—to the pockets between the teeth and the gum. For patients who respond poorly, Keyes prescribes antibiotics such as tetracycline. Surgery is used only when antibacterial measures have failed.

No aspect of the Keyes technique is new, as the originator himself readily concedes. What *is* new is the use of the technique in severe cases of gum disease that previously would have been referred to a periodontist for surgery. Not surprisingly, perhaps, many periodontists strongly object to the Keyes technique as a substitute for surgery in such severe cases. They consider it clinically unproven and potentially more harmful than helpful.

The Keyes technique has attracted dentists in general practice, and increasingly so as preventive measures reduce the income that they previously derived from drilling and filling decayed teeth. These general dentists are tempted to treat cases of severe gum disease that they might previously have referred to a periodontist for surgery. The approach also has obvious appeal for dental patients. Gum surgery, after all, is expensive. The recovery period can be painful. And surgery sometimes leads to still more dental work for cosmetic reasons. Thus, the Keyes technique is clearly an economic threat to periodontists, who depend on general dentists for referrals.

In opposing the Keyes approach, periodontists argue that you must gain access to an infection before you can treat it. While some periodontists concede that surgery may have been used too liberally in the past, they say that in severe cases surgery is still required to eliminate the protective pockets. With the pockets gone, the patient can keep those particular sites clean and help prevent reinfection. Periodontists point out that surgery has proven itself as a long-lasting treatment, while the Keyes technique hasn't. And today's sophisticated surgical techniques, they say, are less painful and can usually produce more cosmetically pleasing results than in the past.

Dentists who endorse the Keyes technique nevertheless accept surgery as a last resort for those cases that don't respond to the antibacterial treatment.

Though new medical treatments usually undergo extensive clinical scrutiny before they're tried out on the public, the Keyes technique seems to have been a notable exception. Many members of the public, and some dentists, embraced the technique even though it had not yet been thoroughly tested in a scientifically controlled clinical study. In fact, recent studies have shown that the antibacterial agents often employed in the Keyes technique are clinically no more effective than properly performed conventional oral hygiene.

RECOMMENDATIONS

Losing teeth is not inevitable. Personal plaque control and professional cleaning are the keys to success in the prevention of gum disease. The following measures have been proven to be successful:

- Brush and floss every day. Thorough brushing usually takes about three minutes. With practice, flossing can also be completed in about the same time.
- Use disclosing tablets or solutions (once a week is the usual recommendation). These products temporarily color existing plaque and show you where you need to work harder at removing it.
- Have your teeth professionally cleaned at least twice a year—more frequently if you neglect your brushing and flossing.
- At each office visit, your dentist or hygienist should give you a refresher course on proper brushing and flossing. Ask for it if you don't get one. Even better, the dentist or hygienist should hand you

a toothbrush and some floss and ask you to demonstrate your skills, so any bad habits can be corrected.

- Don't ignore bleeding gums, which many people consider normal. They are not. If your gums bleed when you brush or floss—or when you don't—you probably have gingivitis, and require professional attention. (Bleeding gums can also be the initial symptom of a bleeding disorder that may require medical investigation.) Note the appearance of your gums. Healthy gums—unless unusually pigmented—should be coral pink. Gums that have a purplish tinge or look puffy are probably inflamed from gingivitis. Other symptoms—persistent bad breath, pus, or teeth that are loose or seem to have shifted position—may indicate severe periodontal disease.

A toothbrush and a length of dental floss are the two most important tools for dental health. Many households add a third tool, the dental irrigator. How effective is it?

According to the *Dentist's Desk Reference*, published by the American Dental Association, an irrigator is no substitute for the brush and the floss. There is no evidence, the *Reference* says, that irrigators remove plaque from the teeth or affect the health of the gums.

On the other hand, the jet of water from an irrigator may help clean out food particles and bacterial irritants that brushing misses. And an irrigator may also be useful for cleaning the teeth around crowns, permanent bridgework, or braces.

20

The Mercury Fillings Scare

The notion that mercury-amalgam fillings are poisoning the populace has been espoused by hundreds of dentists across the country who remove allegedly dangerous fillings and replace them with new ones. Our advice: If a dentist wants to remove your fillings because they contain mercury, close your mouth and watch your wallet.

One hundred million Americans have "silver fillings." The fillings are actually alloys, or amalgams, of silver and several other metals. One of those metals is mercury, which makes up about half the filling. After the puttylike amalgam is inserted, it hardens completely in about one day.

For years, researchers believed that the amalgam released mercury vapor only while it was hardening. But in 1979, University of Iowa researchers found that chewing can release minute amounts of mercury vapor from old fillings. That finding sparked the present controversy over amalgam safety.

IS MERCURY A THREAT?

It's been known for centuries that mercury is a potent poison when swallowed, inhaled, or absorbed through the skin. Prolonged exposure to high levels can damage the brain and nervous system. The classic example occurred in the 19th century, when makers of felt hats dipped material into mercuric-nitrate solution to make the felt easier to shape. In so doing the workers absorbed mercury through their skin and inhaled mercury vapor. Tremors, incoherent speech, difficulty in walking, and feeble-mindedness resulted. The tragedy was rather insensitively immortalized in the phrase "mad as a hatter" and by the Mad Hatter in *Alice in Wonderland.*

Exposure to smaller amounts of mercury vapor can cause less drastic symptoms, including anxiety, insomnia, and minor tremors. Even today, mercury is a hazard for some workers—mainly those in thermometer factories and in plants that use mercury to make chlorine and caustic soda.

Can mercury in fillings cause those or other health problems? "Anti-amalgam" dentists contend that mercury fumes from amalgams can cause problems ranging from depression and multiple sclerosis to fatigue and irritability. Their solution: Drill out the amalgams and replace them with fillings made from other materials. The American Dental Association (ADA), on the other hand, insists that amalgam fillings are safe. Only people allergic to mercury—less than 1 percent of the population—need avoid them, the ADA says.

AMALGAM FILLINGS AND THEIR ALTERNATIVES

Dentists don't make up amalgam with mercury from some perverse love of the stuff. They use it because it's strong and durable. Chewing exerts tremendous force on back teeth—mouthful after mouthful, meal after meal, day after day, year after year. An amalgam filling can withstand those forces for a long time before breaking down. A mercury-amalgam filling usually lasts five to 10 years, and may last as long as 40 years.

The main alternatives to mercury-amalgam fillings are composite resin fillings, which were introduced in the 1960s and are made mainly of plastics. When amalgam fillings are removed because of "mercury toxicity," composite fillings usually take their place. Composites can be mixed to match the color of the tooth, and so are often used for front teeth, where cosmetic considerations may be important. ·

But composites have several drawbacks, particularly in back teeth, where they are subjected to heavy biting pressure. Typically, they have lasted no more than three years. They're also more expensive than amalgam, and teeth filled with composites are less resistant to recurrent decay.

Composites are being continually tested and improved. Research is under way on composites that can be chemically bonded to teeth. Such composites could rival amalgam fillings in durability. CU's dental consultants say that composites strong enough for use in back teeth may become available sometime in the 1990s.

Gold inlays are also sometimes used instead of amalgams. They're durable but cost a lot, both for the gold and for the installation, because they must be preshaped to fit the cavity and then cemented into place. They are not a practical alternative to amalgam fillings.

ASSESSING EXPOSURE AND TOXICITY

Dentists who are looking for a reason to remove amalgam fillings typically use a mercury-vapor analyzer to evaluate the air in the patient's mouth. These devices are customarily used in factories, where they measure the mercury levels in workplace air. Is it appropriate for dentists to use them, as increasing numbers are doing? CU's dental consultants say that use of the mercury analyzer is a scare tactic to get patients to part with their fillings. The device makes it easy for a dentist to contend that a mercury level exceeds occupational standards.

When using the analyzer, the dentist has the patient chew vigorously for 10 minutes, creating heat and friction that maximize the release of mercury vapor. The analyzer senses the mercury contained in about one-half cup of air and multiplies it by 8000. That gives a readout corresponding to the mercury level in a cubic meter of air—about the amount inhaled in an hour. But for the patient, the exposure lasts only a few minutes during chewing—and only a fraction of the vapor may be inhaled. Our consultants point out that most people don't inhale through their mouths while chewing. And even when they're not chewing, most people breathe through the nose, so that inhaled air bypasses any mercury vapor that may be in the mouth. One recent study showed that the analyzer technique tends to produce estimates that are some 16 times higher than the actual daily dose of mercury vapor.

In assessing mercury vapor's effect on health, the key question is: How much actually gets absorbed by the body's tissues? Thomas W. Clarkson, M.D., of the University of Rochester School of Medicine is one of the world's leading authorities on mercury toxicity. He says that a mercury-vapor analyzer can't answer that question.

Clarkson told CU that a person's mercury exposure can best be assessed by measuring the mercury levels in blood and urine. The urine level provides the best measure of "body burden," or long-term exposure to mercury, while the blood level reflects recent exposure. Almost everyone, Clarkson said, has detectable levels of mercury in the urine and blood. The main source of mercury in most people's bodies is the food they eat, seafood in particular.

If dental amalgams really were poisoning people, Clarkson pointed out, the mercury levels in the general population would be at dangerously high levels. That's far from the case. In one study of 1107 people (mainly in the United States), 95 percent had urine levels of mercury lower than 20 micrograms. Adverse health effects appear when the level reaches about 150 micrograms or more, Clarkson said.

If anyone faced a health hazard from mercury fillings, it would be dentists and their assistants. A dentist typically handles between two and three pounds of mercury every year. Skin contact can result in absorption. Careless use and accidental spills can produce significant levels of mercury vapor in the air. Surveys have shown that as many as 10 percent of dental offices have mercury-vapor levels that exceed 50 micrograms per cubic meter of air—the upper limit that the National Institute for Occupational Safety and Health considers safe for eight-hour exposures in the workplace.

Despite their higher exposures, dental personnel aren't being poisoned. Since 1982, the ADA has sponsored a mercury-testing service that measures urine-mercury levels in dentists and dental workers. While average levels are about four times higher than in the general population, they are still well within the acceptable range.

One major reason some dentists are jumping on the anti-amalgam bandwagon can be summed up in one word: fluoride. Largely because of fluoridated drinking water and fluoride toothpastes, the incidence of tooth decay over the past two decades has been cut roughly in half. So some dentists are experiencing a falling-off of business. Removing and replacing amalgam fillings helps to fill that financial hole.

Replacing mercury fillings may cost more than money. Reinvading a tooth—drilling out amalgam and installing a replacement—can increase tooth sensitivity and weaken the tooth. Also, studies show that the very action of drilling out amalgam can produce brief but significant increases in mercury levels in the mouth.

In CU's view, dentists who purport to treat health problems in this way are putting their own economic interests ahead of their patients' welfare. Amalgams have been used for more than 150 years. Except for a few people with a genuine allergy to mercury, CU knows of no reliable studies that show anyone has been harmed by them.

V

WOMEN
and
HEALTH

21

Osteoporosis, Calcium, and Estrogen

Food and drug companies are eager to shore up your bones. Calcium supplements abound, and today's grocery shelves offer a feast of the mineral in products ranging from oatmeal to chewing gum. At breakfast alone, you can toast calcium-fortified bread, wash it down with calcium-fortified orange juice, and even pour calcium-fortified milk on your calcium-fortified cereal.

The calcium craze began innocently enough. In 1984, a panel of scientists convened by the National Institutes of Health (NIH) for a consensus development conference recommended that women obtain more calcium—up to 1500 milligrams (mg) a day. The hope was that additional calcium might help prevent osteoporosis, an abnormal loss of bone most common in postmenopausal women.

In the nutrition arena, even the merest hope has a cash value, especially when that hope is voiced by scientists. Accordingly, when the NIH panel's advice hit the marketplace, it was suddenly transformed into a national health crusade. Images of stooped women, bent and frail from osteoporosis, became a symbol of what could happen to those who failed to heed advertisements for calcium. Sales of calcium supplements soared—from $47 million to $200 million between 1983 and 1987.

Like many nutrition vogues, however, the calcium bandwagon tends to roll over the facts. By the time the NIH held a follow-up conference in 1987, officials found that they had to contend with widespread misconceptions about osteoporosis and calcium.

Despite what ads may imply, loading up on calcium after menopause won't promote a straight spine. And even if it could, some brands of supplements offer little help; they are formulated so poorly that the calcium can't be absorbed by the body. So if you're anxious to avoid osteoporosis, it's important to know what calcium can and can't do for you and how to get what you really need.

OSTEOPOROSIS AND CALCIUM DEFICIENCY

Osteoporosis literally means "porous bone." All adults lose bone as they age, but the excessive loss in osteoporosis makes the skeleton abnormally fragile. An awkward step, a warm hug, or even a strong sneeze may result in fracture.

The disorder afflicts some 15 million Americans, causing at least 1.2 million fractures each year. By age 65, one-third of American women have suffered a vertebral fracture—the kind that contributes to a stoop or "dowager's hump." Osteoporosis also causes an estimated 227,000 hip fractures annually, about twice as often in women as in men. For the elderly, a hip fracture is often more than a painful inconvenience; some 12 to 20 percent of victims die from related complications, such as pneumonia or blood clots in the lungs.

Unfortunately, osteoporosis usually goes unnoticed until it's already severe. By the time ordinary X rays show it, 50 percent of bone mass may be lost. And once bone is lost, it can't be replenished. As of now, the only hope lies in prevention.

The bones reach their peak density somewhere between ages 30 and 40. Then their density starts to decline. One way to minimize the possibility of severe osteoporosis is to start bone loss from a higher setpoint, in effect, by building sturdy bones while you're young. Adequate calcium intake during your twenties and thirties can help do that.

Calcium is the most abundant mineral in the body, accounting for up to 2 percent of an adult's weight. Nearly all of it is found where you might expect—in the bones and teeth. A small remaining fraction in the blood and other tissues plays a critical role in several body processes, including blood clotting, transmission of nerve impulses, hormone action, and muscle function.

Bones are often thought of as inert structures like the steel girders of a building. But they're actually living tissues in a constant state of flux, continually being broken down (resorption) and reformed (accretion). Usually these two factors balance each other. But when calcium is lost from the body or is poorly provided for or absorbed from the diet, resorption gains the competitive edge.

Many Americans—including the overwhelming majority of women—don't get enough calcium. Roughly half of men over age 35 and about 85 percent of women over age 20 don't obtain the Recommended Dietary Allowance for calcium set by the National Academy of Sciences/National Research Council.

The deficit for women is particularly worrisome because nature works against them where calcium is concerned. Women generally have smaller skeletons than men do, and thus lower calcium reserves. Pregnancy, childbirth, and frequent dieting can deplete those reserves further. Hormonal changes that occur at menopause cause women to lose bone seven times faster than men do. So it's important for women to build up calcium reserves before menopause occurs.

Osteoporosis is not only a disease of calcium deficiency, though. It's a complex interaction of genetic, hormonal, nutritional, and life-style factors of which calcium is only a part.

Who Is at Risk?

While there's no way to predict precisely who will and who won't develop the disease, certain factors point to those at greatest risk.

Genetic Factors　Being female is the primary risk. But some women are at higher risk than others. Thin women or women with small bone structures are more susceptible than large, big-boned women. Also, for reasons not entirely understood, the lighter the skin color, the greater the risk. White and Asian women are at much higher risk than black women. Light-skinned, fair-haired women of northern European ancestry are especially vulnerable to the disorder.

Family History　A woman who has a mother, sister, grandmother, or aunt with osteoporosis has an increased chance of developing it herself.

Early Menopause　The earlier estrogen ceases to be secreted by a woman's ovaries—because of surgical removal of the ovaries or an early menopause—the sooner she loses the hormone's protective effect on bone.

Other factors that are more controllable can also influence risk. A sedentary life-style, heavy alcohol consumption, smoking, and excessive caffeine intake all have been linked to the chances of developing osteoporosis. Chronic use of medications that increase calcium excretion may also contribute to bone loss. The main ones include corticosteroids, tetracycline, antacids containing aluminum, and certain diuretics.

PREVENTING OSTEOPOROSIS THROUGH DIET

Obtaining enough calcium in your diet eases the drain on your bones. The National Academy of Sciences/National Research Council sets the Recommended Dietary Allowance (RDA) for adults at 800 mg of calcium daily, an amount calculated to meet the nutritional needs of virtually all healthy people other than pregnant or nursing women. The U.S. Food and Drug Administration (FDA) uses a broader guideline, called the U.S. Recommended Daily Allowance (U.S. RDA), which takes the higher needs of teenagers and others into consideration. The U.S. RDA for calcium, which is the one used in food labeling, is 1000 mg daily.

Manufacturers of fortified foods sometimes go to absurd lengths to sidestep the fact that there are excellent, natural sources of calcium.

"Here's a case for you," says Angela Lansbury, star of the television series "Murder, She Wrote," in a commercial for *Total* cereal. "The case of the missing calcium." Lansbury then proceeds to search in vain for calcium in competitors' cereals. You can find it readily enough, though— in the milk you pour on any of them.

Roughly three-fourths of the calcium in our food supply is in dairy products. Even if you don't drink milk, you can still obtain calcium in a wide range of milk-based products and numerous foods that contain them. Substantial amounts of calcium are found not only in yogurt, cheese, and ice cream, but also in custard, pizza, New England clam chowder, and a host of other foods. You can even consume milk in disguise, adding nonfat-milk powder to sauces, stews, gravies, and casseroles.

Good sources of calcium also include canned salmon and sardines (with soft, edible bones), oysters, almonds, and various green, leafy vegetables. Indeed, many foods contain calcium in at least small to moderate amounts. But unless you're an avid fan of seafood or greens, you'll need some dairy foods on your menu. It takes more than a dozen oysters or a heaping plate of kale, for example, to match the calcium in a single glass of milk.

Furthermore, the calcium in dairy products is readily available to your body—something that can't always be said for other foods, including calcium-fortified products. Milk is fortified with vitamin D, which promotes the absorption of calcium. Spinach and Swiss chard are rich in calcium, but they're also high in oxalates, which bind calcium and hinder its absorption from the intestine.

Nor will you necessarily do better with a calcium-fortified food. Calcium absorption from most fortified foods is as yet untested. If you depend mainly on fortified products, moreover, you may slight other nutrients. A calcium-fortified fruit drink, for example, won't give you the protein of milk. Eating a well-balanced diet is the only reliable way to obtain all the nutrients you need—including calcium.

Although dairy products may be high in fat and calories, your choices aren't limited to ice cream and puddings. Both skim and low-fat milk supply some 300 mg of calcium per cup—at 100 calories or less. At 145 calories, a cup of plain, low-fat yogurt provides 415 mg of calcium. Some cheeses such as Swiss and Muenster do almost as well.

People who are deficient in the intestinal enzyme lactase may have trouble digesting lactose (milk sugar). They may experience gas, bloating, or diarrhea after drinking milk. However, dairy products in which the lactose is already partly broken down—yogurt, buttermilk, and cheeses, for example—often cause no problems. Many people with mild lactase deficiency can also drink modest amounts of milk with a meal. Another alternative is to use a product that supplies lactase such as *LactAid* or *Lactrase.* The product is added to milk to convert part or most of the lactose to sugars that are easier to digest. Pretreated milk is also available in several parts of the country.

PREVENTING OSTEOPOROSIS WITH CALCIUM SUPPLEMENTS

If postmenopausal women lose calcium at a rapid rate, it would seem logical for them to start taking extra calcium at the onset of menopause. But that logic has proved wanting.

Calcium Versus Estrogen

Research since 1984 shows that taking extra calcium *after* menopause has only a marginal effect in slowing bone loss. The primary effect is governed by the action of estrogen, one of two female hormones secreted by the ovaries.

Estrogen is essential for preserving bone in women. At menopause, which normally occurs between ages 45 and 55, the ovaries slow their secretion of estrogen. Women then start losing bone at an accelerated rate. The greatest rate of bone loss in a woman's lifetime occurs during the first five to seven years following menopause. Afterward, bone loss continues but at a slower rate.

A study published in 1987 in *The New England Journal of Medicine* shows that estrogen, rather than calcium, is the key to slowing bone loss in postmenopausal women. The two-year study, conducted in Denmark, compared three groups of women beginning at the time of menopause. One group was treated with estrogen. Another took 2000 mg of calcium supplements a day. The third, a control group, received placebos. The resulting difference in bone loss was dramatic. Bone density in the estrogen group remained constant, while the other two groups lost significant amounts of bone.

Calcium did have a modest effect compared to the placebo. The women who took calcium lost somewhat less cortical bone—the compact bone found in the hip and forearm. However, calcium ingestion had no effect on the spongy, trabecular bone of the spine. Hence, extra calcium taken after menopause would do nothing to ward off a bent spine.

Even though extra calcium offers only marginal benefits after menopause, CU's medical consultants agree with the NIH that taking it is reasonable for women at risk. For those women, any additional edge is desirable. Moreover, for people with normal kidney function and no personal or family history of kidney stones, 1500 mg of calcium a day is safe. For all other adults, the NIH panel's recommendation of 1000 mg daily is a sensible target.

Calcium Supplements

Calcium carbonate is the most widely used form of calcium. If calcium carbonate tablets are not properly formulated, however, they won't provide the calcium you need. In the body, calcium tablets dissolve only in the acidic environment of the stomach. Performance criteria established by the U.S. Pharmacopeia (USP), the nonprofit organization that sets standards for drugs, require at least 75 percent of a calcium tablet to dissolve within 30 minutes—the amount of time it might remain in the stomach. Otherwise, much of the calcium will pass through the body without being absorbed.

Because calcium supplements are considered foods, not drugs, they aren't subject to the same efficacy tests as drugs are under federal law. But a product does have to be what the label says it is. It is illegal to sell a calcium supplement that doesn't provide calcium.

In 1987, Ralph Shangraw, M.D., chairman of the department of pharmaceutics at the University of Maryland School of Pharmacy, tested 80 different calcium supplements. He found that more than half failed to meet USP standards. Consumers Union then performed similar tests on seven nationally available brands of supplements. Four of the seven failed the USP standards.

After Shangraw reported his results at an FDA public conference on osteoporosis, the FDA launched its own field study of calcium supplements. An FDA staff member said the agency will "take action" against manufacturers who fail to meet the USP guidelines for dissolution.

Rather than wait for FDA action, many manufacturers have reformulated their products. But why were so many of the original formulations so inferior? Shangraw offered several reasons. Calcium is bulky. Manufacturers therefore didn't have room for much filler material, such as starch, which helps tablets break up in the stomach. Moreover, companies found that the words "no sugar, no starch" pumped up sales, and many had already removed starch from their formulas. Finally, because calcium is chalky and difficult to swallow, companies often coated pills with shellac. That hinders stomach acids from dissolving the pills. The resulting product tended to act much like a slick pebble.

Other forms of calcium are also available as supplements. Calcium citrate, calcium lactate, and calcium gluconate, for example, dissolve more reliably than calcium carbonate. Their drawback, however, is that the calcium is far less concentrated. Calcium carbonate is 40 percent calcium—compared with 24 percent for calcium citrate, 18 percent for calcium lactate, and only 9 percent for calcium gluconate. That means you'll have to take more tablets—and pay more—for an equivalent amount of calcium.

Another form is calcium phosphate. But tests indicate that it is less soluble than calcium carbonate, suggesting that it is not likely to be a good alternative. Nor are supplements featuring dolomite or bone meal. In the past, some samples of those supplements have been contaminated with lead. "Chelated" calcium tablets are also no bargain. Chelation purportedly improves absorption, but it actually does little more than increase the price.

Clearly, all calcium supplements should be required to meet USP standards. Otherwise, there's no way to be sure the brand you buy will provide calcium in a form your body can use. But even if and when they do consistently meet those standards, you're better off getting your calcium in food.

ESTROGEN REPLACEMENT THERAPY
AND MENOPAUSE

Often the most effective measure for postmenopausal women at risk of osteoporosis is a medical one—estrogen replacement therapy.

Essentially, estrogen replacement therapy involves taking oral doses of estrogen to compensate for the natural decline in its production by the ovaries after menopause. Estrogen can't restore bone mass, so it's not an effective therapy for older women who have already lost a great deal of bone. But if estrogen is started soon after menopause, it can prevent the accelerated bone loss that normally occurs during the first five to seven postmenopausal years. Studies show, for example, that the therapy can reduce the incidence of hip and wrist fractures by 60 percent if begun around the time of menopause.

Estrogen as therapy for osteoporosis is actually one of the hormone's most recent therapeutic applications. Since the 1940s, physicians have prescribed estrogen to afford women relief from the sometimes distressing symptoms of menopause, particularly hot flashes and vaginal atrophy.

Promotional campaigns for estrogen replacement therapy started in the 1960s and, fed by the preaching of a few physicians, flourished for more than a decade. Many menopausal and postmenopausal women were tantalized by the promise that they could remain healthy, youthful, and attractive for the rest of their lives. The promise was summed up in the slogan "Feminine Forever," which was also the title of the book that helped spark the estrogen boom. Millions of menopausal women without severe symptoms were encouraged to take the drug routinely as a cure-all for aging, for the degenerative diseases associated with aging, and for the emotional difficulties purportedly linked with middle age.

Then reports of another side of estrogen therapy began to circulate. Instead of maintaining health and prolonging life, long-term use of estrogen replacement reportedly caused uterine cancer and increased the risk of gallbladder and cardiovascular disease. For many women the dream of agelessness through drug therapy turned into a nightmare of fear and dread. Estrogen usage dropped sharply.

The 1980s brought a renewed interest in a somewhat different approach to estrogen replacement therapy. The culprit behind the seven- to nine-fold increase in the incidence of uterine cancer was found to be not estrogen per se, but rather the use of *unopposed* estrogen—that is, estrogen therapy without concomitant use of the female hormone progesterone. Studies showed that women who received combined estrogen/progesterone replacement therapy had no greater incidence of uterine cancer than did a control group of women. Additional studies have confirmed those results, making combined estrogen/progesterone therapy standard practice.

Estrogen replacement therapy is unquestionably effective and appropriate against certain menopausal symptoms in some women. But which symptoms?

There is no question that menopause is dramatic and undeniable evidence of aging and of the loss of reproductive capability—a double blow for some in a society that worships youth, good looks, and sexuality for everyone. Yet despite physical manifestations of the aging process, femininity and sexuality need not decline as hormones decline. Whether in response to their perceived change in status or to hormonal changes, some menopausal women experience a cluster of psychological symptoms. They may feel nervous, tired, or dejected. They may experience sudden mood changes or suffer from insomnia. How much these emotional manifestations are associated with hormonal changes generally or with the specific distress of hot flashes or vaginal atrophy is not known.

Some menopausal women have hot flashes to a disabling degree. As often as 10 to 20 times a day, a wave of heat, lasting from a few seconds to a few minutes, spreads over the chest, neck, and/or head. It is usually accompanied by a "flush," or increased reddening, and sometimes by drenching sweats. A woman may experience such flashes for only a few months, or they may continue for years. In most cases, they cease within a year or two.

Atrophy of the vaginal lining usually does not develop fully until a decade or so after menstruation ceases, but it can begin sooner. With menopause, vaginal secretions and lubrication may decrease, the vaginal lining begins to thin, and the vagina may become less elastic. Symptoms such as itching, burning, and pain during intercourse may accompany these changes. Urinary discomfort may also occur.

The benefits and risks of treating menopausal and postmenopausal women with estrogen therapy was the subject of a 1979 consensus development conference sponsored by the National Institute on Aging of the National Institutes of Health. The panel's conclusions supported the judicious use of estrogen therapy in women who suffer from severe hot flashes and vaginal atrophy. But, said the report, "There is no evidence at present to justify the use of estrogens in treatment of primary psychological problems." And, according to medical authorities, estrogen replacement cannot prevent or reverse the aging process. (The advisability of estrogen therapy for osteoporosis was left unresolved at the time due to insufficient research data. It has since been shown to decrease the incidence of fractures.)

Estrogen therapy still poses certain hazards. It has been found to promote gallstones, rare liver tumors, and blood clotting factors. The issue of estrogen therapy and breast cancer continues to be debated. Most experts agree that estrogen does not cause breast cancer, although it can promote growth of an already existing breast cancer.

Before a woman starts on estrogen replacement, for whatever reasons, her physician should take a careful history and perform a thorough examination. Liver disease, hypertension, smoking, heart disease, or breast or uterine cancer would likely rule out estrogen therapy.

Because of the risks associated with estrogen replacement, therapy should be reevaluated and discontinued periodically to see if symptoms return. Hot flashes usually need to be treated only for a period of months, according to the FDA, and rarely for longer than a year. Vaginal atrophy may require treatment for a much longer time.

For a woman at high risk of osteoporosis, the benefits of estrogen replacement therapy are now believed to far outweigh the drawbacks. In addition, recent research suggests that taking extra calcium along with estrogen may allow the estrogen dose to be cut in half, further reducing any possible harmful effects.

OTHER MEASURES FOR PREVENTING AND TREATING OSTEOPOROSIS

The spotlight on calcium sometimes obscures the role of other measures to forestall osteoporosis. Among the most important is physical activity, which is vital for preserving bone. The advice here, say experts, is "use it or lose it." But you don't have to run marathons or pump iron to benefit. Even light to moderate exercise can increase bone density.

Not all exercise is equally helpful in building bone. The weightless Skylab astronauts were extremely active and yet suffered bone losses comparable to bedridden people. The best exercises appear to be "weight-bearing" ones—the kind that put stress on the limbs through active movement. Good weight-bearing activities include walking, biking, jogging, aerobics, rope jumping, and practically any active sport that gets you to move around. Swimming, though, is not as effective as other types of exercise because your weight is mostly supported by the water.

If appropriate, reforming your vices can also lower the risk of osteoporosis. Moderating alcohol and caffeine intake and quitting smoking will help your bones as well as the rest of your body.

Other possibilities for the actual treatment of osteoporosis are currently under investigation. Calcitonin, a hormone made by cells within the thyroid gland, enhances calcium deposition in bone; a synthetic version (Calcimar) has been approved for treating osteoporosis. As of this writing, however, evidence that it prevents fractures is limited to a single study. Drawbacks include its cost and the need to administer it by injection. A nasal spray preparation is being developed.

Sodium fluoride, administered by mouth in large doses, has undergone extensive study as a treatment for osteoporosis. Bone density does increase but some experts believe that fluoride bone may not be as strong as normal bone. The prevention of fractures has yet to be demonstrated.

Preventing and treating osteoporosis is clearly more complex than ads for calcium products suggest. If you believe you're in a high-risk category, talk to your physician. If you've already reached menopause, an evaluation of risk factors will indicate whether estrogen therapy or simpler measures are right for you.

22

Drugs in Pregnancy

THE POROUS PLACENTA

Before 1962, generations of physicians were taught the comforting myth that the placenta—the organ within the uterus through which a fetus receives its nourishment—was a sort of guardian angel of the umbilical cord, passing needed nutrients through while holding harmful germs and chemicals back. It was long known, of course, that there were some exceptions. The rubella (German measles) virus, for instance, could be transmitted from a pregnant woman to an embryo in the first three months of pregnancy, causing defects in the fetus. But not until 1962 did many physicians pay serious attention to the possibility that other dangerous substances might be passed from pregnant woman to fetus.

In that year the world was shocked to learn that thalidomide, a drug then commonly prescribed in many countries for insomnia and nervous tension, was in fact a teratogen—a substance capable of producing malformations in a fetus. Thousands of babies born to women who took thalidomide early in pregnancy suffered from phocomelia, or "seal limbs"—so called because foreshortened arms and legs resembling the flippers of seals are the most conspicuous result.

Even today, the world is occasionally shocked to learn of new teratogens. Most recently, the anti-acne prescription drug isotretinoin (Accutane) has been found responsible for hundreds of severe and often lethal birth defects in children born to women who became pregnant while taking the drug. (See page 156.)

Rather than being a barrier to the transfer of drugs from pregnant woman to fetus, the placenta is "a sieve," according to the late Virginia Apgar, M.D., vice president for medical research of the National Foundation–March of Dimes. Apgar said, "Almost everything ingested by or injected into the mother can be expected to reach the fetus within a few minutes." Alcohol, antibiotics, aspirin, barbiturates, sulfonamides, and tranquilizers are but a few of the common, and possibly harmful, substances known to pass through the placenta. Moreover, certain drugs can be found in even greater concentration in the fetal brain, heart muscle, or other organs than in the maternal tissues. In addition, the capacity of the placenta to allow transfer of some drugs seems to increase with the duration of pregnancy.

Much of this information had long been known to the relatively small group of investigators who studied the physiology of the human fetus; but little of their knowledge filtered through to practicing physicians, or even to those responsible for setting the requirements of drug testing. It took the thalidomide disaster to secure wide clinical acceptance of the established facts of fetal physiology. Today physicians assume that, when they prescribe a drug for a pregnant woman, the drug or its breakdown products—with few known exceptions—will also circulate through the fetus.

When pictures of thalidomide babies first hit the front pages, many pregnant women were frightened and immediately discontinued whatever medication they had been taking. Some pregnant women still refuse to take any drugs at all.

We agree that those who are pregnant—and those who are potentially pregnant—should avoid virtually all medication *for the relief of minor symptoms,* especially during the first trimester of pregnancy. However, those who are in need of medical treatment should be guided by their physicians. Pregnant women can have any disease other women have. Tuberculosis, diabetes, infectious diseases such as syphilis and gonorrhea, heart disease, epilepsy—these are but a few of the diseases that, if left untreated during pregnancy, may affect a fetus. Both taking prescribed medicines and refraining from unnecessary medication are important.

A diabetic is a prime example of the type of patient who needs close medical supervision during pregnancy. Diabetics should make arrangements for medical care as early as possible in their pregnancy. Studies indicate that meticulous control of blood sugar, by means of proper diet and use of insulin, can reduce the incidence of fetal abnormalities to the same level as in a nondiabetic population. Those who have been taking oral diabetes medication must switch to insulin for the duration of their pregnancies. These oral hypoglycemics—including tolbutamide (Orinase), acetohexamide (Dymelor), chlorpropamide (Diabinese), tolazamide (Tolinase), glyburide (DiaBeta, Micronase), and glipizide (Glucotrol)—are all now considered unsafe during pregnancy.

THE DANGERS OF DRUGS IN PREGNANCY

"Why don't they first test new drugs on pregnant laboratory animals before permitting pregnant women to use them?" This question was often asked at the height of the thalidomide tragedy, and one of the results of the tragedy has been improvements in animal test procedures.

The FDA guidelines for the evaluation of new drugs for use in pregnancy, announced in 1966, were stricter and better designed than earlier FDA recommendations. The guidelines even specified that a new drug be administered to male animals to check its effect on their sperm cells and their offspring. But as more and more animal tests have been conducted, it has become increasingly apparent that their results may not always apply to humans.

That does not mean that animal tests are worthless for protecting humans. They can serve to arouse suspicion and to remind physicians of the need for caution. But no drug can be considered safe during pregnancy unless it has actually been administered to pregnant women under carefully controlled conditions, and until the babies born to these women have been carefully studied for a period of years to check for defects not diagnosable at birth or during infancy.

Since controlled experiments on pregnant women are quite properly frowned upon, the degree of hazard associated with the vast array of drugs in current use has never been adequately investigated. This is why we caution pregnant women against the use of all drugs rather than just those that have been shown to be harmful.

Some drugs prevent implantation of the fertilized ovum in the wall of the uterus, if used in sufficiently high dosage. They thus act as postcoital contraceptives if their use is begun within 72 hours after sexual intercourse. But a woman who *wants* to become pregnant may use a drug that could have this contraceptive effect, or other as yet undiscovered effects, during the period immediately following conception.

Accordingly, a fertile woman who is sexually active should think of herself as potentially pregnant if she does not use contraceptive measures—and if she would not wish to abort the pregnancy should conception occur. She should discuss with her physician any drug that may be prescribed and at the same time restrict her use of nonprescription drugs.

In this way she would enhance the likelihood of having a healthy baby, should she become pregnant. Most fetal malformations, of course, are caused by factors other than drugs and are not easily avoided. But drug-caused malformations *are* avoidable.

The First Trimester

The thalidomide disaster served to focus popular attention on one kind of drug-related malformation—the kind likely to follow when a drug is taken between the third and twelfth weeks of pregnancy, in the first trimester. During these crucial weeks the fetus begins to assume recognizable form; the basic structures of the brain, heart, arms, legs, eyes, glands, and other organs are laid down day by day. As a result, the malformations produced also vary, depending on the stage of fetal development at which the drug was taken.

The FDA has warned doctors that certain minor tranquilizers—meprobamate (Equanil, Miltown), chlordiazepoxide (Librium), and diazepam (Valium)—should not be prescribed for pregnant patients. Studies have found an association between use of these drugs and fetal malformations, such as cleft lip. The FDA also ordered the manufacturers of these drugs to include a label warning against their prescription during the first trimester.

Examples of other drugs that may be hazardous in the early stages of pregnancy are over-the-counter (OTC) antinausea medications, such as meclizine *(Bonine)* and cyclizine *(Marezine)*. These drugs can cause fetal abnormalities in experimental animals. Although there is no evidence of harm to human beings, pregnant or potentially pregnant women should not use them.

Other well-known medications, including anticonvulsants such as phenytoin (Dilantin), have been found to be associated with an increased frequency of congenital malformations.

All women, especially pregnant women, should be wary of metronidazole (Flagyl), a drug for treatment of a vaginal infection and sold as pills and as vaginal inserts. Studies have shown it to be carcinogenic in laboratory animals; other studies suggest possible genetic damage. Methotrexate, a potent medication that has been prescribed for certain types of cancer as well as severe cases of psoriasis, has been shown to cause fetal malformation. Other anticancer drugs, including azathioprine (Imuran), cyclophosphamide (Cytoxan), and mercaptopurine (Purinethol), when taken in the first few months of pregnancy, have been associated with a high rate of miscarriage.

Vaccination against rubella is inadvisable for pregnant women because of a theoretical risk of fetal abnormalities, particularly when administered during the early stages of pregnancy. Women who are vaccinated against rubella should avoid becoming pregnant for at least three months following vaccination. Women who expect to become pregnant and who are concerned about whether they need vaccination against rubella should be tested for the presence of antibodies to the disease if, as is often the case, they are unsure whether they had rubella in childhood. If the blood test detects the presence of rubella antibodies, the vaccine need not be administered. Many states require this blood test of women who are planning to marry to determine their susceptibility to rubella.

Many other vaccines—including polio, typhoid fever, yellow fever, plague, and cholera—also pose a risk of infection to the developing fetus. If possible, pregnant women should avoid *any* vaccination for three months before pregnancy and during the first trimester. For vaccination after the first trimester, they should consult their obstetrician.

The Second Trimester

Because rubella and thalidomide—the two most publicized causes of prenatal malformations—have been identified as hazards in the first trimester of pregnancy, many people have gained the impression that drugs taken during later stages of pregnancy are harmless. Not so. While malformations arise mostly during the first three months—even before the first menstrual period is missed—hazards of other kinds can occur after that.

One authority has characterized the second trimester as "the great unknown." However, at least two examples of drug-induced damage during the second trimester can be cited. Certain hormones of the class known as progestational agents, formerly prescribed in an attempt to avert miscarriage, sometimes produce masculinizing effects such as enlargement of the clitoris in the female fetus. (Such variations can be surgically corrected.) Substances such as iodides—present in some vitamin and mineral supplements—taken during the second or third trimester may adversely affect the thyroid of the fetus.

Radioactive iodine, often used in the diagnosis of thyroid disorders, should absolutely be avoided during all stages of pregnancy because it can destroy the fetal thyroid gland. For that matter, women should avoid all forms of ionizing radiation, including X rays, during all stages of pregnancy, unless a physician determines that such X rays are warranted despite the possible risk of fetal damage. Pelvimetry by X ray (assessment of the pregnant woman's pelvis prior to delivery) has been replaced by ultrasonography, which utilizes sound waves rather than X rays. When possible, women who are potentially pregnant should schedule any essential X-ray procedures or radioactive isotope tests during the 10 days following the start of menstruation.

The Last Trimester

There are special risks at the end of pregnancy too—and even immediately following delivery of the infant. Several antibiotics may pose hazards, ranging from mild to serious, to the fetus as well as to the newborn baby. Sulfa drugs taken by the mother shortly before delivery may increase the possibility of a certain type of jaundice in the infant. The tetracycline class of broad-spectrum antibiotics may cause permanent staining of the unerupted tooth buds of the fetus. For infections that can be combatted only with antibiotics, penicillin remains safe for use in pregnancy—except, of course, for those allergic to that drug. (Erythromycin appears to be a safe alternative to penicillin—although its safety is less well demonstrated. Cephalexin, another class of antibiotic, is considered safe during pregnancy, but may pose allergic potential to those who are allergic to penicillin.)

Central nervous system depressants, such as barbiturates or narcotics, can slow the breathing of the newborn baby if taken by the mother in high doses during labor and delivery. Anticoagulants, such as warfarin (Athrombin-K, Coumadin, Panwarfin), can cause excessive bleeding in both mother and infant at time of birth and, in some instances when given earlier in the pregnancy, facial deformities in the fetus. Use of indomethacin (Indocin) and aspirin by near-term women has been implicated as contributing to pulmonary hypertension of the newborn.

Are Any Drugs Safe?

To list all the drugs now known or suspected to damage the fetus and newborn baby might lead one to falsely assume the safety of other drugs not yet adequately studied. To conclusively separate safe drugs from dangerous ones, intensive surveillance of birth defects, as well as studies of how pregnant women use drugs—both OTC and prescription—are required. There is also a theoretical possibility that some medications taken by men may affect genetic material in sperm and thus influence fetal development. Researchers have found that a diverse group of known teratogens, when given to male animals only, cause birth defects. These teratogens include alcohol, caffeine, lead, and some narcotics. So far no one is certain how substances administered to (or taken by) males can cause birth defects, or whether they actually would cause such defects in humans. A study made at the University of Vermont discussed several possibilities. For example, drugs could directly damage sperm. Or drugs could be carried in the semen and absorbed through the vaginal walls, thus entering the bloodstream of the female and of the developing fetus. Such theories, though, remain speculative.

A special warning is warranted about the drugs commonly found in the home medicine cabinet. So generally used a drug as ordinary aspirin can interfere with the coagulation mechanism of both mother and baby at delivery. In at least one study aspirin in high dosage has also been associated with an increase in the average length of pregnancy as well as the duration of normal labor. Some learning disabilities have been observed in offspring of laboratory mice given aspirin, although there is no evidence of this in human beings.

No common home remedy, even antacid preparations, should be assumed to be completely safe during pregnancy.

NUTRITIONAL HAZARDS AND OTHER WARNINGS

Vitamin Overdose and Deficiency   Excessive doses of vitamins taken during pregnancy have been known to cause harm to the fetus. If taken in high doses, vitamin C, widely (and falsely—see page 144) publicized both as a cold treatment and as a cold preventive, may cause scurvy in a newborn infant. This is because the large supply of ascorbic acid to which the infant has become accustomed—because of megadosing during pregnancy—is suddenly stopped at labor. High doses of pyridoxine (vitamin B_6) may be associated with withdrawal seizures in the infant. Large doses of vitamin K, if administered near the delivery date, may increase the severity of jaundice in certain infants.

The hazards of excessive amounts of vitamins A and D—which exist for everyone, not just pregnant women—led the FDA in 1973 to set limits on the amounts permitted in OTC vitamin pills: 10,000 International Units for vitamin A and 400 for vitamin D. Physicians could prescribe higher amounts. In announcing the limitation, the FDA commented that among the disorders in which excessive amounts of these vitamins have been implicated were mental and physical retardation. CU and its medical consultants are dismayed that the FDA restrictions were revoked by Congress in 1978.

There is also evidence that dietary *deficiencies* of certain nutrients, such as vitamin C and folic acid, may produce defects in the fetus. Many obstetricians therefore prescribe vitamins in conventional therapeutic dosages for their pregnant patients. But it is important not to exceed these dosages.

Topical Medications A word of caution is also in order concerning medicated salves, ointments, nose drops, suppositories, vaginal creams and jellies, and similar products applied to the skin. Such topical medications may contain substances that can be absorbed through the skin into the bloodstream and thus affect fetal development.

To indicate the nature of such hazards, the FDA issues guidelines for drug labels. For example, the labeling suggested by the FDA for ointments containing cortisone and related steroids is: "Although topical steroids have not been reported to have an adverse effect on pregnancy, the safety of their use in pregnancy has not been established. Therefore, they should not be used extensively on pregnant patients, in large amounts or for prolonged periods of time."

Licit and Illicit Drugs The use of narcotics, hallucinogens, and other mood-altering drugs certainly poses hazards to the fetus. Even the socially acceptable licit drugs—caffeine, alcohol, and nicotine—have been shown to pass the placental barrier. A study conducted by the University of Washington School of Medicine and published in 1973 established a link between maternal alcoholism and birth defects. The researchers concluded that the data point to serious fetal malformations as a possible consequence of alcoholism in the mother.

In 1977 the National Institute on Alcohol Abuse and Alcoholism warned pregnant women that more than two drinks a day may harm their unborn children. The institute has stated that more than 100 studies show a link between a pregnant woman's alcohol intake and malformed or retarded infants. One University of Southern California researcher, recommending total abstinence from alcohol during pregnancy, put the risk of fetal alcohol syndrome defects at 10 percent if a woman drinks between two and four ounces of liquor daily. The National Academy of Sciences/ National Research Council's report, "Alternative Dietary Practices and Nutritional Abuses in Pregnancy," states, "No level of alcohol consumption has been established as safe for the fetus." For years, warning labels on alcoholic beverages were repeatedly proposed and considered by the federal government, but industry pressures prevented adoption of such labeling. As of November 1989, however, every bottle or can of beer, wine, wine cooler, or liquor sold in the United States will be required to carry this warning: "According to the Surgeon General, women should not drink alcoholic beverages during pregnancy because of the risk of birth defects."

Smoking Pregnant cigarette smokers have had ample notice that smoking is associated with an increased risk of fetal and infant mortality. A U.S. Public Health Service report to Congress in 1973 on health implications of smoking reviewed the available research and concluded that about 4600 stillbirths a year in the United States could probably be attributed to smoking. The report referred to a 1972 British study on women who smoked during pregnancy, which showed a 30 percent increased risk of stillborn children and a 26 percent increased risk of infant death within the first few days after birth. However, there is some evidence that women who are able to stop smoking by the fourth month of pregnancy decrease the risk. Smokers, authorities agree, tend to produce babies with a lower average birth weight than do nonsmokers. The Surgeon General's health warnings that now rotate on cigarette packages and advertising include one that reads, "Smoking by pregnant women may result in fetal injury, premature birth, and low birth weight."

Passive Smoking   A study reported in 1982 from the Cleveland Metropolitan General Hospital/Case Western Reserve University showed that when a nonsmoking pregnant woman is heavily exposed to so-called secondhand smoke—that is, smoke from other people—the fetal blood contains significant amounts of tobacco smoke by-products. Although there have been no studies of the clinical effects of such passive smoking during pregnancy, the study's findings are "consistent with the possibility that passive smoking might adversely affect the fetus."

Poor Nutrition   Adequate maternal nutrition is immensely important in pregnancy. Poor nutrition results in lowered birth weights and decreased growth rates for the newborn. And larger weight gains are now recommended for pregnant women that were once thought acceptable. These findings are especially important in light of some current diet fads. We strongly discourage strenuous dieting, especially low-carbohydrate regimens, during pregnancy. These may result in ketosis (the presence of ketone bodies in the blood due to incomplete burning of body fat), which has been linked with subsequent mental retardation in children born to mothers on such diets.

Food Additives   It is extremely difficult to detect such abnormalities as mental retardation and behavioral defects, especially when they are minimal, and to correlate them with ingestion of substances during pregnancy. Some substances may be toxic to the fetus, and these might include a few food additives as well as drugs. Red 2, which was a widely used coloring for foods and beverages (as well as drugs and cosmetics), was judged a possible risk to the fetus, particularly in the period immediately following conception. The possibility that Red 2 might be a cancer-causing agent led the FDA in 1976 to issue a ban on its use. Another additive that may be hazardous during pregnancy is saccharin, which may accumulate in fetal tissue.

Other Hazards Hazards to pregnancy other than those induced by drugs or chemicals are outside the scope of this chapter, with one exception: toxoplasmosis. This parasitic infection, when contracted in pregnancy, may damage the brain and other organs of the fetus. There is evidence that the organism may be transmitted to the fetus when a pregnant woman eats undercooked meat, handles an infected cat, or tends to the cat's litter pan. Infection can occur through inhalation or from hand-to-mouth contamination. Some authorities estimate that about one-third of all adults are immune to toxoplasmosis because of previous undetected infection.

Dietary practices, environmental pollutants, emotional stress—all of these may interact to produce subtle abnormalities, some of which may not even be recognized until many years after birth. There is evidence that some serious abnormalities do indeed take years to develop. One example is the discovery of a hitherto rare type of vaginal cancer in the teenage daughters of women who took diethylstilbestrol (DES) during pregnancy in an attempt to avert miscarriage. Special techniques are required to diagnose this uncommon form of vaginal cancer. It is undetectable by the customary Pap smear test used to diagnose cervical cancer. Any DES daughter should consult a gynecologist knowledgeable on the subject. Studies of DES sons have shown nonmalignant genital abnormalities in some and evidence of impaired fertility in others.

PROPOSALS FOR REDUCING THE RISKS

Correlation between drug use, in its broadest sense, and possible damage to the fetus or the child requires a high degree of suspicion and vigilance on the part of practicing physicians. It also requires that they follow up on any suspected side effect or risk and report to the FDA what they believe to be an adverse drug reaction.

Competent authorities have made many suggestions for further reducing the risks of drugs in pregnancy. Here are five proposals CU supports.

1. Increased Understanding About Drugs in Pregnancy on the Part of Physicians and Their Patients. Shortly before the thalidomide disaster, a study made in California showed an incredible number of drugs—nearly 11,000 in all—actually prescribed by physicians to 3072 women whose pregnancies began during the 12-month period ending March 31, 1961. Only 244 of the patients (7.9 percent) went through pregnancy without a prescription; and only 563 (18.3 percent) had only one drug prescribed; 617 women received more than five drugs each; 121 women received 10 or more, and a few received 20 or more.

These totals did not include self-prescribed drugs, OTC drugs, and drugs prescribed before pregnancy that patients continued to take during pregnancy. Some prescriptions contained more than one drug ingredient. The actual number of risks was considerably higher, because one drug alone may be effective and safe but may be rendered ineffective or harmful when taken at the same time as one or more other drugs. Some of the drugs prescribed were no doubt essential for the health or well-being of the patient or her unborn baby. But many others were superfluous.

No one really knows how much more cautious physicians have since become when they write prescriptions for their pregnant patients. But the evidence is not encouraging. Based on several studies, it has been estimated that 90 percent of all pregnant women take at least one prescription medication during the course of their pregnancies.

CU supports educational programs about drugs in pregnancy—for physicians and the general public alike. Doctors should be strongly encouraged to consider the risks when prescribing or advising medication for a pregnant—or a potentially pregnant—patient. And if medication is warranted, a patient should be warned to take drugs only in prescribed amounts and for specified durations. There is urgent need for clearly worded warnings and guidelines to be prepared for distribution to pregnant women by physicians, pharmacists, clinics, and other health agencies.

2. **International Cooperation in Testing.** Following the thalidomide disaster, the United States, Canada, Great Britain, France, Germany, and other countries tightened up animal test procedures. In many respects, however, foreign test requirements remain less strict than the FDA guidelines. Even so, certain clinical drug studies, performed abroad under guidelines similar to FDA standards, may be acceptable as part of the FDA's review process preliminary to approval of a new drug application.

3. **Primate Tests.** Most new-drug tests are now performed on pregnant rats, mice, and rabbits. Would tests on monkeys or other primates more closely related to humans secure results more valid for pregnant women? No one really knows. The FDA "encourages" tests on pregnant monkeys but does not require them; they are rarely run because they are so expensive. A large-scale research program designed to determine whether primate tests are worth the extra cost is thus CU's third recommendation.

4. **Reporting of Adverse Effects.** The thalidomide hazard was unmasked when physicians in West Germany and Australia noted a sudden, startling increase in infant malformations of a type encountered only rarely before. Improved procedures for reporting events of this kind have been instituted. It is unlikely that if another drug like thalidomide comes along its teratogenic effects would be overlooked until 5,000 or 10,000 had been afflicted.

The recent experience with birth defects caused by the anti-acne drug isotretinoin (Accutane) demonstrates how much sooner teratogenicity is likely to be detected. In this case, the animal tests revealed the drug's potential for causing birth defects even before it was marketed. But a warning label and physician education effort proved inadequate to prevent another tragedy—although on a smaller scale than that caused by thalidomide. Between 1982 and 1986, the number of babies born with defects caused by Accutane during pregnancy was anywhere from 62 to 1300—depending on whether you accept the manufacturer's estimates (based on actual reported cases) or the FDA's (based on extrapolation from the data). In 1988, an expert advisory committee to the FDA recommended that distribution of the drug be severely restricted to make it more difficult for young women to obtain. (See pages 155–56 for more on Accutane.)

While the Accutane experience indicates improvement in the system for catching drug hazards during pregnancy, the problem has not been solved. The next teratogen to be discovered may not produce a dramatic and readily recognizable pattern of otherwise rare defects. The next new drug may produce mental retardation, for example, or premature birth, or some other already common misfortune. If so, it could affect thousands of babies without revealing itself; such afflictions could easily go unnoticed among the countless similar cases already occurring. What is needed as an alerting mechanism is continuous registry of the occurrence of all malformations and other perinatal conditions in an entire population. Then, if some common condition is seen to be increasing in frequency, a search for causes can be promptly undertaken.

In the United States, the Birth Defects Monitoring Program, coordinated by the Centers for Disease Control in Atlanta, keeps watch over approximately one million births yearly, based on computer data compiled from records of some 950 participating hospitals. Limitations are built into the monitoring system, however, since hospital records of newborns often may not include such information about the child's mother as age, number of previous pregnancies, and medications taken during pregnancy.

Although the program would undoubtedly discover any disaster on the scale of the thalidomide tragedy, it probably cannot detect the causes of small clusters of birth defects. The system does not provide the kinds of information necessary to establish a clear connection between birth defects and maternal drug use.

Authorities on surveillance of birth defects believe some relatively simple changes would improve the effectiveness of monitoring programs. Procedures for linking birth defects with maternal factors could probably be strengthened if terminology were standardized, hospital records were kept in a uniform fashion, and hospital admission records for infants required information about the mother.

5. **Patient Package Inserts.** Before any drug can be marketed, the pharmaceutical firm responsible must secure FDA approval of a "package insert" or "product information circular," which lists precautions and contraindications as well as indications, dosages, and other important data. One difficulty with package inserts as a means of alerting busy physicians to a drug's possible hazards for pregnant women has been the question of format and type size. The information about pregnancy could once have been a few words buried in a thousand words or more of small type on other subjects—an unlabeled item under "Warnings" or "Contraindications."

In 1979, new FDA regulations for prescription drug labeling required specific information about a drug's potential for possible harm to the fetus. Listed under "Precautions," a special subsection on pregnancy is now mandated for all drugs absorbed systemically and likely to affect the fetus. Such drugs are labeled according to one of five pregnancy categories—A, B, C, D, or X:

A. The possibility of fetal harm is remote. Adequate and well-controlled studies in pregnant women have shown no increase in risk of fetal abnormalities.

B. The possibility of fetal harm appears remote. Either animal tests have failed to demonstrate a risk to the fetus and there have been no human studies, or animal studies have shown some evidence of risk, but well-controlled tests with pregnant women have provided contrary evidence.

C. Benefits outweigh potential risks. Either there have been no animal or human studies demonstrating adverse effects, or animal studies have shown teratogenic effects but there have been no adequate and well-controlled studies in humans.

D. There is potential hazard to the fetus. Positive evidence of risks based on adverse reactions in humans must be weighed against potential benefit from the drug.

X. Fetal abnormalities have been demonstrated.

Labeling must also include information on the drug's nonteratogenic effects, labor and delivery, and nursing mothers.

All of the above regulations about improving package inserts deal with material addressed to physicians. CU believes that patients have a right to direct access to information about the implications of drug usage. Manufacturers have included FDA-approved package inserts prepared especially for patients in some prescription drugs. Information sheets on many other drugs are made available for physicians to distribute to their patients.

Of course, package inserts are not a panacea; the Accutane tragedy demonstrated that many women—and their physicians—may still overlook or ignore such warnings. Nevertheless, CU endorses patient package inserts and would like to see them extended to cover other medications, starting with those likely to be hazardous during pregnancy. In 1981, however, the Reagan administration withdrew federal support from the FDA-supervised patient package insert program, despite strong protests from CU and other consumer organizations.

RECOMMENDATIONS

We have stressed the drug factor in malformations and other problems of fetuses and newborns because something can be done about it right now, both by patients and by health professionals. But it is also important to keep the drug factor in proper perspective.

The great majority of malformations and other unfortunate outcomes of pregnancy are caused by factors other than drugs. And the number of infants with major congenital abnormalities is not the only crucial factor. Drug hazards should be stressed not because the ill effects are so numerous or so likely to occur, but because when they do occur they can be so devastating. And in most instances, the hazards of drug use can be so easily avoided. Pregnant women who follow the precautions listed below and whose physicians use ordinary prudence in prescribing for their patients can be assured that the risks and side effects of drugs in pregnancy will be minimized.

We recommend that the following cautions be observed by pregnant women, as well as by fertile women who engage in sexual intercourse without contraception.

• Do not take any drug unless there is a compelling medical need for it. Be especially careful in the first trimester of pregnancy and just before delivery.

• If there *is* a medical need, and if your physician prescribes a drug to meet that need, take it only in the amounts and at the times specified. Do not increase or reduce the dosage; do not discontinue usage sooner or continue it longer than directed. Remember that fetal health can be adversely affected by your failure to take a needed drug as well as by your use of unprescribed medication.

• A number of drugs exert their adverse effects during the first weeks following a missed menstrual period—the weeks when you may be wondering whether you are pregnant. Therefore, if pregnancy is a possibility, discontinue all self-prescribed remedies when an expected menstrual period fails to occur, and recheck with your doctor concerning drugs previously prescribed for you. (A simple blood test can now determine pregnancy on the very first day of a missed menstrual period.) If you are trying to become pregnant, be sure to inform your doctor if a drug is prescribed for you.

• During pregnancy and also during the time you may wish to become pregnant, curtail the use of OTC "home remedies," as well as nonessential prescription drugs. Even common self-prescribed medicines, such as aspirin, should be taken sparingly, if at all.

• Mothers who breast-feed their babies should continue to avoid the use of medications as much as possible. Numerous drugs taken by the mother are excreted in her milk and reach the nursing baby. If a nursing mother is prescribed a medication, she should tell her physician that she is breast-feeding her baby.

• Interpret the term *drugs* broadly to include many things besides oral preparations and injections—for example, lotions and ointments containing hormones or other drugs that may be absorbed through the skin, and vaginal douches, suppositories, creams, and jellies.

VI

AIDS
and
BLOOD-BORNE
DISEASES

23

AIDS

THE FEAR EPIDEMIC

By any measure, AIDS is a frightening disease. It is physically devastating, incurable, and lethal. And it is spreading at a menacing pace. Fear and misconceptions about AIDS, however, have spread faster than the disease itself.

Federal health officials stress that the AIDS virus has spread almost exclusively by three routes: by sexual intercourse, through blood contact (contamination with or transfusion of infected blood or blood products), and from an infected pregnant woman to her fetus or newborn. The only other known instances in which the virus was transmitted, say officials, involved artificial insemination or organ transplants from infected donors.

But many people remain unconvinced. They fear that casual personal contact with an AIDS victim—a handshake, a sneeze, a drink from the same glass—might lead to infection. A child with AIDS attempting to attend school can throw a community into a frenzy. An AIDS patient returning to work may find coworkers deserting the job in protest.

In short, anxiety about AIDS has itself become epidemic. Part of the problem is that AIDS is a new disease—mysterious in its origin and initially baffling in its symptoms and cause. But the impression that scientists are groping amid a welter of unresolved questions is misleading. A vast amount of critical knowledge has already been gained about AIDS, and more is being learned all the time.

The epidemic first surfaced in the late 1970s, when rare cancers and uncommon infections began appearing in a number of gay (homosexual) men. Those illnesses were linked with a severe deficiency in the body's immune-defense system—a disorder initially called GRID, for Gay-Related Immune Deficiency. As late as mid-1981, gay men were still the only known victims in the United States, creating the impression that AIDS arose from something exclusive to that group.

By 1982, when the name became AIDS, for "acquired immune deficiency syndrome," the first currents of fear jolted the health-care community. The number of AIDS cases was rising geometrically, and the disease had appeared in two more groups—intravenous drug users and hemophiliacs. Not only did the pattern imply an infectious agent, but the disease was now affecting three of the principal groups vulnerable to hepatitis-B infection—a viral illness that's also an occupational hazard among health workers.

AIDS would subsequently prove to be much less contagious than hepatitis B, partly because the number of hepatitis-B virus particles in blood is up to a billion times greater than the number of AIDS virus particles. But no one knew that in 1982. Nor was it known that the AIDS virus doesn't penetrate intact skin or the linings of the respiratory and digestive tracts—and thus could not be transmitted by such things as a kiss on the lips, a cough, or food prepared by a person with AIDS.

With the number of cases doubling every six months, medical personnel on the front line became increasingly fearful for their own safety. That fear soon became evident to the public at large, helping to confirm impressions that a virulent plague was loose in the land. As public fear of the threat grew, scientific understanding of the disease advanced rapidly.

By mid-1984, three independent research teams in the United States and France had conclusively identified the virus that causes AIDS. Discovery of the virus—now designated "human immunodeficiency virus," or HIV—immediately opened new avenues of research into every aspect of the disease. Investigators have already deciphered the genetic code of the virus in search of ways to attack it. Others probing for clues to therapy have explored its crippling effect on the immune system.

For epidemiologists, who investigate the incidence, transmission, and patterns of disease, identification of the virus was the indispensable handle for a powerful new tool. It meant that a test could now be developed to detect individual exposure to the virus, information vital for deeper insight into the epidemic and its spread.

ELISA: TESTING FOR EXPOSURE TO AIDS

By 1985, a simple, inexpensive blood test for detecting exposure to the AIDS virus had been developed and approved for use. Called ELISA (for enzyme-linked immunosorbent assay), the test detects antibodies produced by white blood cells in response to the presence of the virus. Developed primarily to screen potential blood donors (see Chapter 24), ELISA has also served as a versatile research tool, greatly facilitating analysis of the epidemic's path.

Before ELISA, it was difficult to trace the spread of the virus. There was no practical way to detect it in people without symptoms, who represent the largest number of those infected. By mid-1988, about 65,000 cases of AIDS had been reported to the U.S. Centers for Disease Control (CDC). An estimated 325,000 people had AIDS-related complex (ARC), a term used to describe a condition that includes (in addition to laboratory evidence of immunodeficiency) swollen glands, recurrent fever, weight loss, or a combination of those symptoms. When persons with ARC develop any one of a number of opportunistic infections (or Kaposi's sarcoma), they are considered to have developed AIDS.

An estimated 1.6 million to 3.2 million additional people may be infected with the virus but have no symptoms of illness. Although their blood reveals antibodies to the virus—as determined by two consistently positive ELISA tests and a more sophisticated (and costly) confirming test called Western blot analysis—they may have no other laboratory or clinical signs of disease. Most public-health officials estimate that 30 to 50 percent of those people will ultimately develop full-blown AIDS.

With a practical means of detection in hand, researchers began probing areas previously obscure. For example, how fast was the virus spreading to the general population—or among intravenous-drug users, or gay men? Was it infecting family members who had no sexual contact with a victim in the home? Were some sexual practices riskier than others? Since 1985, a wealth of new information has become available to address those questions and others.

Some of the findings are uncompromisingly bleak. Among high-risk groups, the AIDS virus is cutting a widening swath of infection, particularly in areas that have already borne the brunt of the epidemic, such as metropolitan New York and San Francisco. The infection is also spreading among young adults in inner-city minority groups, especially black and Hispanic intravenous-drug users and their sexual partners. One analysis of blood tests administered to some 300,000 military recruits found the rate of infection in blacks to be four times that in whites.

Federal health officials have predicted that the cumulative total of AIDS cases could reach 270,000 by 1991, with 179,000 deaths. Most of those will be people who are already infected with the virus, the officials said.

The grim projections of unfolding tragedy have overshadowed all other emerging information about the epidemic. But there has been another side to the news. An increasing number of epidemiological studies now point to an unmistakable conclusion: The reassurances from health officials about casual contact with AIDS patients are well founded. As CDC director James O. Mason, M.D., put it, "This is a very difficult disease to catch."

Transmission appears to require not only direct insertion of the virus into the bloodstream but also a substantial dose of the virus—much more than could be transmitted by casual contact. Indeed, a consistent pattern in people who become infected is frequent or severe exposure to the virus.

Even in sexual intercourse—the primary route of infection—the virus does not appear to spread easily. Like most sexually transmitted diseases, AIDS is strongly associated with a highly active sex life and multiple partners.

HOMOSEXUAL TRANSMISSION

Among gay and bisexual men, the disease first appeared in those with extremely large numbers of sexual partners—a lifetime average of over 1000 partners, according to one early epidemiologic study. It's not known whether multiple sexual contacts raise the risk simply by raising the odds that a person will encounter the AIDS virus once, or by some process in which the body's defenses are worn down (perhaps through exposure to other sexually transmitted diseases), or both. All that's known for sure is that having a large number of sexual partners raises the risk.

Now that the virus is more prevalent—and the odds of catching it (among people at risk) are higher—the average number of sexual partners reported by people who contract the disease would be *far* less than 1000. No precise numbers, however, are available.

A key factor in the rapid spread of the virus among gay and bisexual men is the practice of anal intercourse, probably because the surface membranes and blood vessels of the anal canal are vulnerable to small fissures or tears during intercourse. Such tears may allow virus carried in semen to gain entry into the bloodstream of the receiving partner. The risk of viral transmission is especially high for the partner accepting penetration (receptive anal intercourse). In one six-month study examining transmission of the virus in gay men, a University of Pittsburgh research team found receptive anal intercourse to be the major risk factor in infection. At the outset, none of the men showed any evidence of AIDS virus in their blood. After six months, however, antibodies to the virus were found in a number of the subjects, especially among men who had had two or more sexual partners. In that group, men engaging in receptive anal intercourse had 16 times the infection rate as those having no anal intercourse.

As yet, there's no scientific evidence that sexual practices other than anal-related sex lead to AIDS-virus transmission in gay men. However, only a few large studies have compared the effects of different sexual practices.

One such study was conducted by University of California researchers over a two-year period for the San Francisco Men's Health Study. The California investigators examined infection rates among some 800 gay or bisexual men with different sexual histories. No difference in infection rates was found between those who engaged solely in oral-genital sex and those who had no sexual partners at all.

The California researchers concluded that the risk of AIDS-virus transmission by oral-genital contact was minimal. But they cautioned—as did the Pittsburgh group—that their findings did not prove that sexual activity other than anal intercourse posed no risk among gay men. They pointed out that their results were based on a relatively small number of observations and could not completely exclude the possibility of transmission by oral-genital sex.

Indeed, caution has been the watchword among public-health officials offering preventive advice. Since more than 90 percent of AIDS cases have occurred in gay or bisexual men and intravenous-drug users, the message to those high-risk groups has stressed avoiding any possible risk. One drawback of that approach, however, is that it makes AIDS appear easier to catch than it actually is. Some public-health workers, for example, warn against deep kissing involving exchange of saliva. But there's no evidence that the virus is transmitted that way (see pages 239–40).

HETEROSEXUAL TRANSMISSION

In contrast to oral sex or deep kissing, vaginal intercourse is clearly an important route of infection. The AIDS virus can be spread by either a man or a woman during intercourse.

On a relative scale, vaginal intercourse appears to be less effective in spreading the virus than anal intercourse, and less contagious from female to male than the reverse. As yet, the risk of transmission in a single act of vaginal intercourse is unknown. But current evidence suggests that frequent or long-term sexual exposure with an infected partner or partners is an important factor in transmission.

As of mid-1988, about 4 percent of newly diagnosed AIDS cases in the U.S. can be traced to heterosexual transmission. A large number of the victims are spouses or long-term sexual partners of AIDS patients or other high-risk individuals, particularly intravenous-drug users. Another large segment includes immigrants from Haiti and central Africa, where the virus spreads mainly by heterosexual intercourse.

Some confusion initially surrounded the status of Haitians, who were once listed as a separate risk group for AIDS. Epidemiologists have since found that the infection rate is not high among Haitians who are long-term U.S. residents. It's high, though, among recent immigrants with a history of venereal disease or sexual contact with prostitutes. In both Haiti and central Africa, infected prostitutes are an important factor in the spread of the virus among heterosexuals.

Reports from central Africa also show that AIDS is concentrated among urban people who are very sexually active. The average AIDS patient had more than 30 sex partners a year, including frequent contacts with prostitutes.

Overall, heterosexual spread of the infection often involves multiple sexual exposures to the virus. Even under these circumstances, however, infection is far from automatic. In a number of studies based on antibody tests, 50 to 65 percent of the regular heterosexual partners of patients with AIDS or advanced AIDS-related illness have shown no evidence of the virus in their blood. And among the wives or regular sex partners of hemophiliacs with AIDS, 90 to 95 percent were not infected.

The fact that such prolonged sexual exposure often fails to cause infection certainly argues against fears that a bathtub, toilet seat, or the air around an AIDS patient could pose a threat.

Public-health officials generally recommend using condoms during anal or vaginal intercourse and oral-genital sex to reduce the risk of AIDS-virus transmission. CDC investigators, after evaluating many studies from around the world, concluded that barrier contraceptives—condoms, spermicides, and diaphragms used with spermicides—are effective in reducing the risk of sexually transmitted diseases, including AIDS. Lubricants, if used, should be water-based; petroleum products can damage latex.

One lab experiment demonstrated that the AIDS virus can't penetrate an intact latex condom. Another showed that a common spermicide, nonoxynol-9, inactivates the virus and kills the white blood cells that carry it. (Nonoxynol-9 is the spermicide in many contraceptive jellies and foams, and the active ingredient in the contraceptive sponge *Today*.)

BLOOD-TO-BLOOD CONTACT

The rapid spread of the AIDS virus among intravenous-drug users fosters the impression that the virus is highly infectious. Actually, some common practices among addicts who use needles are what make them especially vulnerable. And while there is some evidence that gay people have modified their risk behavior, drug abusers have not.

In addition to the frequency of injections—at least daily in many users—intravenous-drug addicts often share their needles and syringes. Indiscriminate sharing of injection paraphernalia has become common at drug "shooting galleries," where addicts go to rent or share equipment. "Often, the same needle will be used for up to 50 injections until it is no longer usable," reports Peter Selwyn, M.D., medical director of a drug-treatment program for addicts at Montefiore Medical Center in the Bronx, New York.

The risk of contamination is multiplied by another practice—drawing blood back into the syringe so that any remaining drug can be flushed out of the syringe and into the vein. If an addict is infected with the virus, a significant dose of it may be transmitted to the next sharer. In short, intravenous-drug use is an extremely effective way of acquiring a blood-borne disease—even one as difficult to contract as AIDS.

Some people have proposed that government agencies should make sterile needles and syringes available to intravenous-drug users, either free or at cost. Facing the threat of an AIDS epidemic in 1984, the Amsterdam (Netherlands) Municipal Health Service adopted such a plan. It appears to be working. The number of addicts using intravenous drugs has not increased, and more addicts than ever have been motivated to enter treatment for their addiction. Similar programs have since been initiated in Sweden, Great Britain, France, Italy, and Australia.

Such proposals in the United States have generally met with strong opposition. In 1988, the first attempt at a free-needle program was made in Portland, Oregon; it stalled when insurance coverage was refused. New York City began a similar program the same year. Yet even advocates of the idea recognize it as a stopgap measure. They emphasize the need for more drug-treatment centers and a multifaceted approach to the problem. But an epidemic often demands swift action. Cheap, clean needles and syringes would at least reach the inner-city battleground where AIDS has hit hardest and where the real war on drugs is being fought—and lost.

The experience of health-care workers, meanwhile, provides a striking contrast to the epidemic among intravenous-drug users. Seven separate studies in the United States and England have examined the outcome of needle-stick and other exposures among health workers caring for AIDS patients. Approximately 1500 people—nurses, physicians, medical students, technicians, and laboratory workers—were studied to determine whether their exposures had resulted in infection. Most of the exposures were needle-stick injuries from instruments that had just been used for an AIDS patient. The rest were direct exposures of a mucous membrane, such as a splash of infected blood into the eye or nostrils.

Despite the large number of exposures, only five of the 1500 workers developed AIDS-virus antibodies in their blood. Those five had experienced a severe exposure, such as a deep injection wound or a puncture from a grossly contaminated large-bore biopsy needle. None of the workers who had direct exposure of mucous membrane to blood or other body fluid developed infection.

Hemophilia, a genetic disorder marked by the absence of an important clotting factor, results in repeated bleeds, often into joints. Transfusions of blood products can correct the bleeding temporarily. Before routine screening of blood and blood products for the AIDS virus was initiated in 1985, many hemophiliacs became infected. Since then, the risk has been virtually eliminated.

CASUAL CONTACT: HOW AIDS IS NOT TRANSMITTED

Detection of the AIDS virus in saliva in 1984, and subsequently in tears, sparked immediate public concern. But further research has shown that the virus is rarely present in either. When it is, the quantity is minute—probably too low, say most public-health experts, to play a role in infection. Nevertheless, as a precaution, they still warn against deep kissing with an infected person and advise special procedures for eye-care and dental personnel, who are constantly exposed to tears or saliva.

No such precautions apply to contact with drinking glasses, eating utensils, eyeglasses, and the like. All evidence shows that the risk from such items is nonexistent. The same is true for a typical friendly kiss.

Some parents of young schoolchildren also fear that a bite from an infected classmate might transmit the virus. Here again, the concern is unwarranted, experts at the CDC say. The amount of virus in saliva—if any—is considered too minuscule to cause infection, especially in a single instance of biting.

There is no evidence that the virus can be transmitted by food or by any variety of insect. Nurses who have administered mouth-to-mouth resuscitation to AIDS patients have not become infected. Nor have children attending school with hemophiliac classmates who were infected. But possibly the strongest evidence that the virus presents no threat in casual contact comes from studies in families.

If AIDS could spread through casual contact, a patient's home would be a likely breeding ground of infection. The close personal environment of a family household would offer ample opportunities for spreading the virus.

It hasn't happened, however. Studies in U.S. households and among families in Europe, Haiti, and central Africa have all produced the same result. No instance of transmission has occurred among anyone who wasn't the sexual partner or newborn infant of an infected person.

The most comprehensive study is an ongoing, long-term investigation being conducted jointly by the CDC, Montefiore, North Central Bronx Hospital, and Albert Einstein College of Medicine. In 1986, the research group reported its evaluation of 101 people living in households with 39 AIDS patients. None of the 101 household members were sexual partners of the patients, but all lived in close personal contact with the infected person for periods ranging from three months to four years.

"Most of the families in this study were poor and lived in crowded conditions," the researchers reported. "A high percentage of household members assisted the patient with bathing, dressing, and eating." There was close personal interaction, and substantial sharing of household facilities and items likely to be soiled with body secretions. Some of the household members used the same razors and toothbrushes as the patient. Many shared the same combs, eating utensils, plates, and drinking glasses. More than 90 percent used the same toilet, bath, and kitchen facilities as the patient, and 37 percent shared the same bed. Most also engaged in affectionate behavior with the patient, including hugging and kissing on the cheek or lips.

Except for one child infected at birth, all of the 101 households examined were found to be free of any sign of AIDS virus in their blood. The researchers concluded that transmission of the virus through ordinary personal contact "appears to be minimal or nonexistent in the household setting."

The research group has continued its investigation since that report. As of the spring of 1988, it had completed examinations of more than 200 family members in more than 75 households, including reexaminations of the original subjects. None (except the one child) showed evidence of infection.

Similar findings were recently reported from central Africa. A research group in Kinshasa, Zaire, investigated whether the same results reported among household members in Europe and North America apply under conditions common in the developing world.

"Unlike living conditions in the United States and Europe," said the report, "living conditions in households in Kinshasa are more likely to include environmental factors favoring person-to-person transmission of infectious agents." Such conditions, the report said, included "crowding, lack of modern sanitary systems, and substantial numbers of mosquitoes and other arthropods."

The study, which evaluated 204 household members of AIDS patients, found no evidence that the virus was spread by ordinary personal contact. The researchers concluded that transmission by nonsexual personal contact "appears to be very rare, if it occurs at all."

The Kinshasa group also suggested what many American and European epidemiologists have come to realize, with profound relief: Since the AIDS virus isn't spreading in the home, transmission by casual contact in workplaces, schools, or similar settings will probably never occur.

24

Is the Blood Supply Safe?

Almost two-thirds of all blood used in transfusions goes to surgical patients. Those who receive it usually face lower risks from transfusion than from anesthesia and surgery. But, then, surgery *sounds* risky. Getting blood does not—at least it didn't until the discovery that the AIDS virus could be spread through blood transfusions. For the first time, many people realized that the nation's blood supply was vulnerable.

Yet blood can harbor a variety of infectious microbes besides the AIDS virus. And even perfectly acceptable blood can cause problems in some recipients.

By far the most crucial factor in a transfusion is the proper match of blood types. Human blood is classified into four major types: A, B, AB, and O. Blood with red cells of one type will commonly contain antibodies against some or all of the other types. Transfusing the wrong type of blood can cause serious reactions—in extreme cases, shock, kidney failure, and even death.

Fortunately, the blood-banking system safeguards against such mix-ups. Blood banks type and label blood as soon as it's collected. Before hospitals use blood, they cross-match it with the recipient's blood to make sure the two are compatible. Minor incompatibilities sometimes escape the cross-matching process, but serious reactions from them are uncommon. A person who receives blood for the first time has only a one-in-10,000 chance of an adverse reaction. If it happens, that reaction is usually chills and fever.

A much greater risk arises from infected blood. Blood-borne parasites and viruses can cause malaria, hepatitis, and AIDS, as well as less familiar diseases. Cytomegalovirus, for example, gained brief but worldwide notoriety in 1981 for complicating Pope John Paul II's recovery after a transfusion he received for blood loss from a gunshot wound.

Blood banks can't test for all infectious organisms; there are just too many. Instead, banks rely partly on a series of questions to screen out potential carriers. One set of questions focuses on identifying people most likely to be carrying the AIDS virus. Among those are gay men, intravenous-drug users, hemophiliacs, recent immigrants from Haiti and certain parts of Africa, and people who have engaged in prostitution anytime since 1977, as well as their sexual partners.

After the initial screening, blood tests provide the second line of defense, especially against AIDS. The ELISA test, or "enzyme-linked immunosorbent assay," detects an antibody to the AIDS virus, indicating that the prospective donor has been exposed to infection. The test, which is now performed on all donated blood, is designed for maximum sensitivity, so that any questionable blood will test positive. While this results in many false-positive readings, it makes ELISA highly effective as a screening tool.

If the ELISA test is positive, repeat tests are done. Unless two repeat tests are negative—indicating that the first test was a false positive—the blood is withheld from the blood supply and ultimately destroyed. Blood that's positive on two ELISA tests is also subjected to a more sophisticated and expensive test, the Western blot. If that test is negative, the bank assumes the ELISA results were in error (but even so, the blood is destroyed). If the Western blot test is positive, the bank notifies the donor that he or she has been exposed to the AIDS virus, and typically offers to arrange counseling.

Despite its sensitivity, ELISA may not detect AIDS-tainted blood if a recently infected donor is just beginning to make antibodies to the virus. It usually takes from a few weeks to about three months after exposure to the virus for antibody levels to reach the point of detection. However, such "false negative" results are rare. As of mid-1988, federal health officials had identified only 16 cases of AIDS-virus infection that can be traced to transfusions received since April 1985, when ELISA tests were adopted for blood donors.

THE GREATER THREAT: HEPATITIS

While public fears about the blood supply have focused on AIDS, hepatitis poses a far more common threat—and one that can be just as deadly. The American Red Cross has estimated that the chances of receiving AIDS-contaminated blood in a transfusion are less than one in several hundred thousand. By contrast, the chances of receiving hepatitis-contaminated blood may be as high as one in fifty.

There are three forms of hepatitis, two of which present little, if any, threat to blood recipients. In hepatitis A (infectious hepatitis), the virus is blood-borne only during the acute phase, when the victim is already becoming sick, and most unlikely to be giving blood. Another form, hepatitis B (serum hepatitis), was virtually eliminated from the nation's blood supply by an accurate screening test developed in 1972. But a third form, designated non-A/non-B hepatitis, infects roughly 2 percent of all those who receive a blood transfusion.

There is as yet no treatment for non-A/non-B hepatitis. At its worst, the virus can cause severe liver disease, including cirrhosis and cancer. Of the people who develop acute hepatitis, one in three will progress to a form of chronic hepatitis. And one in 20, according to some estimates, will ultimately develop cirrhosis.

Screening tests for carriers of non-A/non-B hepatitis have been non-specific—they haven't been able to detect the presence of the virus itself, only signs that it might be there. In 1986, faced with an unacceptably high hepatitis rate among transfusion recipients, blood banks reluctantly began using two marginal tests for non-A/non-B hepatitis. They hoped each would compensate for the deficiencies of the other, together picking up 40 to 60 percent of the contaminated blood. In short, the tests have been wrong as often as right, allowing some hepatitis-contaminated blood through and causing good blood to be thrown out.

In 1988, one group of researchers reported that the virus responsible for non-A/non-B hepatitis had been isolated for the first time. A specific antibody test to detect carriers of the disease may soon become available.

DONATING YOUR OWN BLOOD TO YOURSELF

The only blood that's virtually risk-free in a transfusion is your own. In emergencies, of course, medical personnel have to depend on blood from the public supply, since the risks associated with blood transfusions pale before the immediate need to save someone's life. But less than 20 percent of transfusions are required for emergencies, reports the American Association of Blood Banks (AABB). In cases of elective surgery, physicians often can help patients arrange for an *autologous transfusion*—one that uses the patient's own blood.

Patients who want to use their own blood have two options. They can donate and store a few pints of their blood before surgery. Or, in special cases, the surgeon can use a procedure called "intraoperative salvage" to recycle the blood lost during surgery. (Intraoperative salvage is used mainly in large medical centers for heart and chest surgery, which often involve heavy blood loss. The procedure requires special equipment and people trained to use it.)

Using your own blood virtually eliminates the risks associated with blood transfusions. Infectious diseases are no longer a threat: You can't give yourself something you don't have. Nor need you worry about allergic or immunologic reactions. Your immune system will gladly accept your own blood. The American Medical Association, major blood-banking institutions, the U.S. Food and Drug Administration, and the National Institutes of Health all recommend that you donate your own blood before elective surgery. That recommendation does not extend, however, to speculative blood banking—paying a blood-storage company to freeze some of your blood "just in case."

The Wrong Way . . .

Several blood-storage companies have cropped up around the country in recent years. One of them, Idant Laboratories in New York City, which has run a frozen-sperm bank for years, initiated a new type of "employee benefit" by signing agreements with Warner Communications and IMS International to provide blood-storage services for all of their employees.

It's expensive to store your blood on the chance that you might some-day need it. Between charges for typing, testing, freezing, and storing your blood, you can easily pay over $500 a year. There's another charge for withdrawing your blood from the bank (plus transportation costs)—but don't worry, it's highly unlikely that you'll ever need it.

The chance that any one person will need blood in the next year, or even the next three years (the longest that red blood cells can be stored frozen), is slim; and in emergencies, people who have paid to store their blood may still have to depend on the public supply. Frozen red cells must first be thawed, then washed by hand to remove dead cells. That takes at least 90 minutes. Then there's the problem of getting the blood to you—no small feat if, say, you've been in a car accident hundreds of miles from the blood center.

S. Gerald Sandler, M.D., of the American Red Cross says that blood-storage companies are capitalizing on the fact that blood banks can't guarantee that someone receiving blood won't contract a disease such as hepatitis or AIDS. But, says Sandler, "the alternative doesn't guarantee that people who need blood will be able to use the blood they have stored."

An unpublished study by the Red Cross reveals how seldom frozen blood is used—or needed. The Red Cross maintains a supply of frozen red cells for people with rare blood types, the largest supply of frozen blood in the nation. They surveyed 3000 people in their rare-donor registry to gauge how the blood was being used. Only 20 people had used any of the stored blood; and in every case, the Red Cross concluded, an aware donor could have donated his or her own blood in the weeks before surgery. In no instance were the frozen cells used in a traumatic bleeding incident to save anyone's life.

. . . and the Right Way

With a bit of foresight, physicians can usually schedule elective surgery to allow their patients enough time to donate a few pints, or units, of blood beforehand. Studies published in the journal *Transfusion* and in *The New England Journal of Medicine* report that two-thirds of patients who predonated their blood needed no additional blood from the public supply. Those who couldn't donate all they needed still reduced their risks by limiting their exposure to the blood of others. Another study, published in *The Journal of the American Medical Association,* examined an autologous blood program used for orthopedic patients at a Florida hospital since 1976. Over a 10-year period, 95 percent of the blood used was autologous. Even though a few patients needed additional units from the public supply, the hospital had encountered no instance of hepatitis symptoms among patients who took part in the program.

The benefits of autologous transfusions extend beyond the patient. Safe blood is also reassuring to surgeons. Because of the risks associated with ordinary transfusions—especially from several different donors—surgeons tend to be stingy with blood that comes from the public supply. For example, blood plasma (the fluid part of the blood) is ideal for certain types of plastic surgery because it both replaces fluids and aids in blood clotting. But the surgeon often winds up substituting a saline solution because the benefits of the plasma don't justify the risks. If the plasma is the patient's own, however, the surgeon will gladly use that rather than salt water.

Using your own blood also helps ease the burden on the public supply. Red Cross officials estimate that they lose about 10 percent of their potential donations because either the donor or the donor's blood doesn't pass their screening tests. But such tests are waived for autologous blood. Every unit you predonate represents a unit saved for the public supply.

Autologous transfusions are dramatically underused. Joseph Bove, M.D., as chairman of the AABB's committee on transfusion-transmitted disease, estimated that less than one percent of the transfusions in the United States before 1987 used a patient's own blood. The study published in *The New England Journal of Medicine* reported that out of 20,640 units of blood used in transfusions at 18 hospitals, only 193 were autologous units. The authors concluded that fully two-thirds of the patients in the study could have avoided blood from the public supply by predonating their own.

Autologous transfusions are probably underutilized because they are more work for everyone involved. The vast machinery it takes to get the public blood supply's 12 million units of blood annually from donor to hospital to patient runs surprisingly smoothly. But a John or Jane Doe who wants to donate and get back the *same* units of blood adds an extra cog to the system. Enough Does and the system has to be reworked or it may grind to a halt.

In recent years, almost every major medical organization in the United States has endorsed the use of autologous transfusions. As the practice becomes more common, hospitals and blood banks will have little choice but to adjust.

How Autologous Transfusion Works

To gain the advantage of presurgical donation, you should ask your physician as soon as elective surgery is scheduled whether you'll need a transfusion. If you can use your own blood, you'll need time to make donations. Your surgeon should make the necessary arrangements with the community or hospital blood bank.

The main requirement for predonating blood is that you be in reasonably good health. Many people who are ineligible to donate to the public supply—because of age, weight, or medical history, for example—can store blood for themselves. The only thing that absolutely precludes storing blood for your own later use is an active infection, such as the flu.

Blood-donor guidelines normally recommend that people give blood no more than once every eight weeks, which allows a wide margin of protection against anemia. But that limit is waived for autologous donations. You can usually store up to one pint per week for four to six weeks (depending on hospital policy), with the last unit being taken as late as 72 hours before surgery. (Blood counts should be checked along the way to make sure that nothing worse than mild anemia develops.)

The six-week maximum arises because that's the limit on how long blood can be stored fresh. Although red cells can be kept frozen for up to three years and plasma for a year, many hospitals do not use frozen blood in their autologous programs because it's more expensive.

Your body restores the lost fluid volume within a few hours of donating blood, but red cells are replenished more slowly. Not everyone can donate blood weekly without becoming anemic. Not everyone has to: The average amount of blood required in a transfusion is only 2 or 3 units. Even patients who donate only part of what they need still reduce their risk.

Most hospitals charge the same for your own blood as for blood from the public supply. A few charge less. The Red Cross reports that some of their banks in urban areas tack on a surcharge of about $25 for the cost of special handling. As long as you are storing blood for upcoming surgery at your physician's request, most insurance companies will cover any extra costs, including those of getting to and from the blood bank. Note, however, that insurance coverage applies only to blood that's actually transfused, not to units beyond what you need.

Some patients who can't donate their own blood turn to friends or family members rather than to the public supply. Although some banks will take such "directed" donations with a physician's consent, most discourage the practice. There's no evidence that directed donations are any safer than blood from the public supply. Indeed, many experts suspect such donations could be less safe.

Directed donations bypass one of the safeguards in blood banking—

anonymity. Someone who donates blood anonymously has no incentive to disguise the fact that he or she may be in a high-risk group for transmitting disease. Some friends and relatives, on the other hand, might find it preferable to donate than to explain how they happen to fall into one of the high-risk groups. If the hepatitis or ELISA test is positive, moreover, only the donor is notified. The patient may not learn that the blood has been rejected until he or she arrives for surgery.

Another common misconception—especially since the emergence of AIDS—is that giving blood might somehow expose the donor to infection. Impossible. The equipment used is sterile and disposable. There is absolutely no risk of contracting AIDS or any other disease when you donate blood.

VII

MIRACLES
of
MODERN
MARKETING

25

Foods, Drugs, or Frauds?

According to the House Subcommittee on Health and Long-term Care, quackery was a $10 billion business in the United States in 1984, and growing at an alarming rate. Bogus "nutrition supplements" represent a significant part of the business.

Many nutrition supplements sold in health-food stores are claimed to treat or prevent a variety of diseases, delay aging, restore pep, and work many other wonders. These claims are made despite lack of scientific proof—and often despite plenty of scientific proof to the contrary. Health-food store owners may not know that the claims are unproven—or disproven.

You won't find these claims on the labels of the bottles that line the shelves. Instead, the treatment-and-prevention allegations appear elsewhere: in pamphlets stacked nearby, in books and magazines available for browsing or purchase, or in "bag stuffers" given away at the checkout counter. Often, buyers have no way of knowing whether this literature comes from the manufacturers of the products.

For manufacturers and distributors of nutrition supplements with inflated claims, it makes good legal sense to keep the products separate from information about their claimed benefits. If a label merely says "take 2 tablets 3 times daily as a dietary supplement," the product is arguably a food supplement—and thus not subject to the federal laws governing drugs. But a therapeutic claim—say, "take 2 pills 3 times daily for relief of arthritis"—legally qualifies the product as a drug and subjects it to regulation as such by the U.S. Food and Drug Administration (FDA).

A drug, under the law, is a product "intended for use in the diagnosis, cure, mitigation, treatment or prevention of disease in man or other animals." A drug can be legally marketed if it has been approved by the FDA, or if it is "generally recognized as safe and effective." If a drug meets neither of these criteria, the FDA can seize it, prevent the company from marketing it, and seek criminal penalties.

Many nutrition supplements bear a disclaimer saying that they are "not intended to replace the services of a physician." But the claims made for them, and the manner in which they are marketed, send the opposite message to buyers.

Some unproven remedies, as detailed later in this chapter, can cause serious injury because they contain toxic ingredients or contaminants. Many others, though innocuous themselves, encourage the victims of serious diseases to medicate themselves, substituting ineffective substances when effective treatments exist.

NUTRITIONAL SUPPLEMENTS: DRUGS IN DISGUISE

In recent years, many companies have begun playing the drugs-as-foods game. To get acquainted with some of them, CU created its own health-food store in 1984. We operated our store in two different states under two different names. That way, we could be sure all the products we ordered were shipped in interstate commerce, and thus subject to federal regulations. We could also learn whether health claims were being made for the products by the manufacturers or distributors. If so, the products are legally considered drugs—even if the claims never appear on the labels.

We contacted more than 70 companies and asked for their catalogs and product information. We chose our products and sent back the order forms, along with requests for additional literature to help explain the products' uses.

In addition to more than 300 products, much literature was bestowed on us during the five months we ran our store: "Dear Retailer" letters from manufacturers explaining why their products should be prominently displayed; numerous catalogs filled with detailed product descriptions; dozens of free fliers, brochures, "fact sheets," and bag stuffers to help us "increase sales dramatically." Some of this literature did indeed contain astonishing medical claims.

Our health-food store's products and accompanying literature, of course, were not sold to consumers. Instead, they were evaluated by a seven-member panel of medical and legal experts. The panel comprised four attorneys specializing in health and health-fraud issues, a specialist in internal medicine on the faculty of a major university medical center, a nutritionist, and a pharmacologist on the faculty of another major university medical center.

The panel evaluated one or two products from each company. For each product, the panelists made a judgment about whether the product was legally a drug; whether it was known to be effective for its claimed purpose; whether it posed a direct hazard to the user; and whether it posed an indirect hazard by encouraging users to abandon other forms of therapy. Many of the products were judged indirect hazards. A few were judged direct hazards—substances that could cause harm to the user.

The final judgment the panelists made was whether the manufacturer or distributor was violating the federal Food, Drug and Cosmetic Act. New drugs must have FDA approval as being safe and effective before they can be marketed. New drugs marketed without FDA approval are considered illegal.

The panel also looked at whether the product could be legally considered "misbranded." A product is misbranded if the label doesn't provide adequate directions on how to use the product for its advertised purposes, or if the labeling (which includes any literature used in the distribution of the drug) is false or misleading in some way.

In the panelists' unanimous opinion, 42 of the 70-plus companies offered products that violated both major provisions of the Food, Drug and Cosmetic Act: They were unapproved new drugs *and* they were misbranded. The products of a few of these companies have been seized by the FDA. One company has been criminally prosecuted by the FDA. Most, so far as we know, have never been the subject of any FDA enforcement action.

Our panel judged five products to be the worst of the entire bunch. A sixth product, glandular concentrate, was found to be legally marketed—but particularly disgusting.

Liquid Citrus Bio-Flavonoid Complex If the panel had given an award for the most outrageously illegal claims made for a product, the award might have gone to *Liquid Citrus Bio-Flavonoid Complex,* manufactured and distributed by Bio-Botanica Inc., of Hauppauge, New York.

Bio-Botanica sent our store numerous copies of a flier entitled "Bio-Flavonoids and You!"Although the product *label* was clean, the flier indicated that *Liquid Citrus Bio-Flavonoid Complex* can help people with the following maladies: "herpes sores ... easy bruising or hemorrhaging ... diabetic cataracts ... capillary oozing during surgical procedure ...

abnormal clumping of red blood cells and blood platelets . . . cancer-producing processes . . . excessive inflammation . . . abnormal uterine bleeding . . . allergy symptoms in children . . . cystitis toxicity . . . capillary bleeding caused by anti-coagulants . . . menopausal symptoms."

Bio-Flavonoids are a mixture of organic chemicals found in citrus fruits. Discovered in the 1930s, they were called "vitamin P" for a short time—until researchers found they were not essential for humans. (A vitamin, by definition, is. See Chapter 14.) They have not been proven useful for treating any human maladies.

Padma 28   Many of our health-food-store products, while not harmful in themselves, were found to be hazardous because they might prompt users to forgo effective medical treatment. Of all the products reviewed, our panel singled out *Padma 28* as the most dangerous such "indirect hazard."

The *Padma 28* tablets purportedly contained 22 herbs prepared "in accordance with the principles of Tibetan herbology." An ad placed by Padma Marketing, the product's Berkeley, California, maker, boasted that "*Padma 28* produces results in treating angina pectoris and PAO [peripheral arterial occlusion]." A flier the company sent to our store touts *Padma 28* not only for angina and PAO but also for "disabilities of old age, especially in relation to reduced circulation, such as senility, poor memory, and depressed energy levels," and for "poor circulation in general, producing cold feet, numb or antsy feeling in the arms and legs, stiffness of the joints."

The panel considered the claim that *Padma 28* relieved angina "highly dangerous." Panelists said that anyone using *Padma 28* for angina attacks instead of seeking help for the underlying heart problem could be making a fatal decision. Depending on the amount consumed, *Padma 28* could also represent a direct hazard. One of its ingredients is the herb aconite, which is poisonous. How much aconite do you get with *Padma 28*? The label (unlike labels for approved drugs) didn't say.

Meganephrine   "Dear Friends," the letter to our store began, "Nutritional specialty products are among the most effective agents that can be used in the prevention and treatment of coronary heart disease, stroke and related life-threatening complications." The letter was from Arteria Inc., of Concord, California. Arteria products are notable for having scientific-sounding names such as "Essential Mucopolysaccharides," "Acetylcholine Releasers," and "Electrolyte Replenisher."

Our panel reviewed claims for an Arteria product called *Meganephrine.* "This nutritional supplement," the company said on the order form, "is especially designed to offset adrenal insufficiency and also raise serum noradrenaline levels." Does anyone really need a higher noradrenaline level? We doubt it: Noradrenaline is made not only in the adrenal glands but also in various nerve endings throughout the body. Deficiencies have not been described in the professional medical literature.

The panel considered *Meganephrine*'s claims dangerous. The key claim was that the product cures adrenal insufficiency. Treatment of this rare disorder requires the services of an endocrinologist and judicious use of corticosteroids. Anyone who takes *Meganephrine* and gets away with it almost certainly never had adrenal insufficiency. A person who actually has the disease and who uses this product instead of the usual hormone replacement therapy could become seriously ill within a day or two and might even die.

Meganephrine's ingredients come mainly from animal innards. The recipe for each capsule was "250 mg Adrenal; 40 mg Hypothalamus; 50 mg Pituitary; 100 mg Medulla concentrate; 250 mg Tyrosine (an amino acid)." These ingredients are no more helpful than a hamburger.

DMSO A brochure put out by Life Extension Products, of Fort Lauderdale, Florida, advertises "DMSO in the Treatment of Cancer Patients." The ad claims that DMSO could be "one of the most effective anticancer agents known," that it "has the properties desired in any cancer drug" and has been "used successfully" with chemotherapy.

The ad does contain one fact—that DMSO "is capable of passing through body tissue taking other products with it." But that fact makes DMSO a substance that could be directly, as well as indirectly, hazardous.

DMSO is an industrial solvent. The FDA has approved a purified form solely for the treatment of interstitial cystitis, a rare bladder disease. But otherwise, DMSO has not been shown to alter the course of any other disease. Nevertheless, proponents of DMSO therapy claim miraculous relief from a variety of ailments, notably arthritis. Despite public-education efforts by the FDA, many people obtain industrial-grade DMSO from nonmedical sources and attempt to use it medically.

After receiving our DMSO from Life Extension, we read the instruction sheet on "Use of DMSO in the Treatment of Cancer." We could take it orally ("use one ounce of 100% DMSO mixed with three ounces of orange juice") or rectally, as a retention enema ("mix one ounce of 100% DMSO with three ounces of water").

DMSO could prove fatal, according to CU's panel, if used as a retention enema. As the Life Extension ad stated, DMSO does "take other products with it" as it "passes through body tissue." In the rectum, these "other products" might include bacterial toxins that DMSO could carry through the intestinal wall and into the bloodstream. For a person who is already weakened by cancer, the effect of the absorbed toxins could be life-threatening.

Another recommendation in the instruction sheet advised diabetics who use insulin to "decrease the insulin intake by 40–50% during the DMSO treatment" and to consume sugar "regularly with the DMSO doses." For some diabetics, following this advice could lead to diabetic ketoacidosis, a dangerous complication that could lead to coma and death.

Rheumoid In the literature we received, NF Physicians Formula Inc., of Portland, Oregon, called itself "An organization of health-care practitioners dedicated to the promotion of wellness." The company's 50-page catalog listed 292 diseases and conditions, ranging from Alzheimer's disease and angina pectoris to seizures, stroke, and warts. The product guide, or "Clinical Repertory," matches each ailment with the "nutritional substances" it says are effective in helping to rebalance the patient.

Our panel looked at one such "nutritional substance," called *Rheumoid*. The *Rheumoid* tablets contained seven herbs, an amino acid (L-cysteine), and potassium. An NF Physicians Formula information sheet described *Rheumoid* as "a safe and effective alternative to the arthritis drugs currently in use"—a claim that disturbed the panel because it could encourage people to turn away from effective medications. In addition to arthritis, *Rheumoid* was touted for back pain, discopathy, osteomalacia, osteoporosis, and scoliosis.

Our panelists found that NF Physicians Formula was just one of many companies that purport to market products only to "health care professionals." Chiropractors appear to be the biggest customers. Federal law prevents chiropractors from writing prescriptions for FDA-approved drugs, so companies such as NF Physicians Formula offer them the chance to "prescribe" something. Chiropractic journals we reviewed are full of ads for unapproved remedies.

Gland Concentrates Long a staple of quack health spas and clinics, "raw gland concentrates" have become a health-food fad. A seller's pamphlet explained, "The theory is that like cells help like cells." So swallowing capsules of raw adrenal concentrate, for example, will supposedly "bolster the function" of your own adrenal glands.

The FDA considers glandular supplements to be inert, dried glandular meats, which are digested like other meats and have no other value. The agency says it has acted against thyroid gland supplements, which might be used by people who believe they were a substitute for prescription thyroid products. But the FDA told CU it cannot act against other organ-type products, such as dried liver, kidney, and the like, unless a drug claim is made.

CU's panel reviewed "raw glandulars" marketed by several companies. Because manufacturers generally don't make therapeutic claims for these products, the panel considered them to be legally marketed foods. But the panel suggested that some glandulars be tested for bacteria. We sent our 13 glandular preparations for lab analysis, and got back some interesting results.

Manufacturers often boast that they process the glands at low temperatures. For example, the labels on glandulars from Biotics Research Corp. (Houston, Texas) said, "Dehydrated at low heat (40°C./104°F.) to preserve associated enzyme factors." Such relatively low temperatures also help preserve something else: contaminating bacteria.

An expert at the U.S. Pharmacopeia considers 100 bacteria per gram an unacceptably high level. Of the 13 products tested, seven had unacceptably high bacteria levels. In the worst product, one gram had a standard plate count of 6.5 *million* bacteria per gram. These included 24,000 coliform bacteria—intestinal bacteria whose presence indicates that hazardous intestinal organisms may also be present. The next-worst product had "only" 4900 bacteria per gram, including 1100 coliform bacteria.

It's immaterial whether these glandular products are legally considered foods or drugs. Those with high bacterial content are adulterated and hazardous and, in our view, should be barred from distribution.

THE DUBIOUS DISTRIBUTORS

Another dimension to the health-fraud boom is the person-to-person peddling of nostrums within multilevel sales schemes. It's easy to become a distributor. Just visit any of the "health expos" held regularly in major cities around the country. You'll find dozens of booths filled with enthusiastic representatives explaining how you can improve your health and make good money at the same time. Thousands of Americans have become distributors for these multilevel marketing organizations selling nutrition supplements.

Distributors buy products wholesale and sell them retail to relatives, friends, and neighbors. But to make big money as a distributor, you must usually sign up others to work as distributors under you—and help your distributors get people to work, in turn, for them. You get a percentage of all sales made by your "downline." This marketing plan is commonly known as a "pyramid scheme."

At the same time that we operated our health-food store, one CU reporter trained as a distributor for several nutrition-supplement businesses. It was a frightening experience.

In one typical initiation, our undercover reporter visited an established distributor for one such organization. Nancy (not her real name) ushered our fledgling distributor into her apartment living room. Lining one wall were four shelves filled with pill bottles and boxes. Nancy explained what the products would do.

"This one," she said as she plucked a bottle off the shelf, "cures diabetes." She said she knew of cases in which diabetics taking the product had been able to come off insulin. The company can't make claims like that on the label, she said, "or the FDA would get after us."

Another item was for cancer—both prevention and cure. That product, she said, "works with the immune system" and for that reason can also cure AIDS. She personally knew three patients who took the stuff and "every one has gotten over AIDS." Can I actually tell people that? our novitiate asked. "Theoretically, you shouldn't make medical claims," Nancy said. "But I said it right off. It'll cure AIDS. Because it's true. Face to face, you can say anything you want."

Emphasize testimonials, Nancy advised. Recite cases in which the products successfully conquered disease. The new distributor's own experience with a product will also help convince people, she said. "You can say that it helped you if it did. Or even if it didn't."

Initiation rites into these distributorships vary. But the deceptive sales strategies they teach are much the same.

WHY THE FDA DOESN'T CRACK DOWN

Health fraud is thriving today for several reasons. Throughout the nation, there is a keen interest in health, whether you call it fitness, wellness, or prevention. Many legitimate businesses and products ride this wave of interest—and the quacks do, too.

The fear of pesticides and other chemicals—good or bad—has added to people's interest in healthful, "natural" products. Also, many people view modern medical practice as too impersonal or too profit-oriented. That distrust has also played into the quacks' hands.

The FDA didn't create the health-fraud boom. But, clearly, fighting health fraud ranks low among the agency's priorities. In 1988, the agency had a budget of more than $477 million. Of that, approximately $2.4 million, or only about one-half of 1 percent, went primarily to combat quackery. Such FDA efforts against health fraud have consisted chiefly of public-education activities and civil actions (primarily injunctions and seizures of merchandise). In 1987, the agency recommended 12 seizures, one injunction, and no criminal prosecutions. The FDA has largely abandoned criminal prosecutions as an enforcement tool in health-fraud cases.

Some FDA officials have maintained that criminal cases are always more expensive and time-consuming than civil cases. But others disagree. They say that simple, carefully chosen criminal cases need not cost more—and can have a strong deterrent effect. These officials contend that the civil actions favored by the FDA don't deter. White-collar criminals, they say, view a product seizure as merely a cost of doing business.

In its earlier days, the FDA used criminal prosecution considerably more frequently than in recent years.

At the turn of the century, dangerous patent medicines were flourishing: sinus powders containing cocaine, "soothing syrups" sweetened with opium and morphine, painkillers loaded with toxic acetanilid, cancer cures spiced with radium. To halt abuses in the sale of medicine and to combat the even larger problem of adulterated food, Congress passed the Pure Food and Drug Act. But the 1906 law didn't give much enforcement authority to the agency that later became the FDA.

A 1937 tragedy caused Congress to give the FDA the enforcement power it had previously lacked. A small Tennessee drug company concocted a liquid variant of sulfanilamide, a legitimate medicine widely used to treat bacterial infections. This "Elixir Sulfanilamide" contained a then-untested toxic solvent, diethylene glycol. It killed at least 107 people.

That disaster led to the Food, Drug and Cosmetic Act of 1938. For the first time, manufacturers had to prove their drugs were safe before marketing them. The law also removed a major enforcement hurdle. Until then the FDA, to obtain criminal convictions, had to prove fraud—that a company *intentionally* committed violations, such as making false therapeutic claims about its product. Under the new law, the FDA could win convictions merely by showing that the violations had occurred.

Over the next 25 years, the FDA put some notable quack promoters out of business—and often behind bars. By 1957, the FDA reported that there were "more defendants . . . serving jail sentences for false curative claims than at any time in FDA history."

In 1961, FDA Commissioner George P. Larrick boasted of his agency's progress against health fraud in general and nutrition quackery in particular: "The Food and Drug Administration has had considerable success in combatting food quackery in the courts. There have been some heavy fines and some prison sentences. . . . Such actions have had a marked deterrent effect."

Compare that to a 1982 speech on the same subject, prepared by Arthur Hull Hayes, then the FDA Commissioner: "'Okay,' you may be thinking, 'if [quackery] is such a big problem, what is the FDA doing about it?' The answer, I'm afraid, is not much. We are . . . simply overmatched."

The FDA knows about the many products and marketing schemes that violate the law. But the agency no longer vigorously enforces the law. In the fight against health fraud, it seems that the FDA has pretty much thrown in the towel.

One authority has suggested that the FDA's deemphasis of quackery stems indirectly from another drug disaster—thalidomide, the tranquilizer that produced birth defects in the children of women who used it during pregnancy (see Chapter 22). The thalidomide tragedy prompted Congress to push the FDA into much closer supervision of prescription drugs. In 1962, Congress passed the Kefauver-Harris Amendments to the 1938 law. The amendments required that drugs must be proven not only *safe* (as required by the 1938 law) but also *effective* before the FDA could allow them on the market.

The amendment vastly increased FDA responsibility for dealing with legitimate drugs—both prescription and over-the-counter. The agency had also taken on increased responsibility in the realm of food safety. With these major new duties, the FDA's priorities shifted sharply.

In 1984, following a four-year review of health fraud, the House Subcommittee on Health and Long-term Care issued a 250-page report that particularly criticized the FDA's efforts. It found that the agency, "once a formidable force in controlling quackery," no longer met that description. "Considering the thousands of known quack remedies marketed each year, the potential for harm, and the billions [of dollars] lost yearly, [the FDA's] effort and the relatively few prosecutions generated by the FDA seem minimal at best," the report concluded.

The subcommittee introduced three bills that gave nutrition-supplement quacks quite a scare. The measures would have promoted consumer health education, increased criminal penalties for quackery, and created an interagency Strike Force to enforce those penalties. Vigorously attacked by those whose livelihood depends on peddling nutritional supplements as drugs in disguise, all three bills died.

26

Generic Versus Brand-Name Drugs

In 1983, a group of New York State legislators tried to save consumers money by changing the prescription forms used by physicians. Under their proposal, patients in New York would receive a generic drug from pharmacists unless the doctor prescribed a brand-name drug and wrote "dispense as written" on the form. A prescription drug marketed under its generic name can cost half the price of the same drug sold under a brand name—the name given it by the company that held the original patent.

Three of America's largest drug companies—American Home Products, Bristol-Myers, and Hoffmann-La Roche—sent key New York legislators a "Memorandum in Opposition." It featured aerial photos of two modern "major pharmaceutical manufacturers" played against a ground-level photo of "a New York City generic manufacturer." The latter focused on a garbage-strewn vacant lot. "We would appreciate your contrasting their facilities," the memo said, "and question whether you believe [they] can uniformly produce identical drug products."

That was the opening salvo in yet another round of a long war waged by the makers of brand-name drugs against the generic drug firms that compete with them. The brand-name companies dominate a prescription-drug market worth $25 billion a year as of 1987. They barrage legislators, physicians, pharmacists, and consumers with an unrelenting message: Generic drugs are low in quality and may harm you. Few distortions in the history of commercial propaganda have cost consumers more money than that one.

WHO MANUFACTURES WHAT

The firms that make brand-name drugs are called "innovator" drug companies. There were 59 such U.S. companies in 1986; by 1988, the number had jumped to 92. Each of them devotes millions of dollars a year to developing new drugs and ushering them through a long testing and

264

approval process. When an innovator's drug is finally approved by the U.S. Food and Drug Administration (FDA), the company gives it a brand name such as Valium or Inderal and then spends millions more promoting it. As a reward for its investment, the innovator earns a patent that protects the drug from competition for a number of years, usually at least a decade. Until the patent expires, the innovator may license other companies to produce the drug—with FDA approval—under their own brand names. Once the patent expires, any pharmaceutical company can apply for FDA approval to produce its own version of that drug and market it under the drug's "generic" name—diazepam rather than Valium, for example, or propranolol rather than Inderal.

Most generic drugs are manufactured not by seedy factories operating next to garbage dumps but by the very same companies that develop brand-name drugs. Indeed, in 1986 the 59 innovator drug companies manufactured about 80 percent of all generic drugs, in addition to their brand-name products. Some 300 smaller pharmaceutical companies scrambled for the rest of the generic market.

More than a dozen companies now produce generic diazepam to compete with Valium, which is made by Hoffmann-La Roche. Those manufacturers include not only generic companies but also two of the largest innovator firms, American Cyanamid and Warner-Lambert. The tablets differ from Valium in color and shape, and in the inactive "excipients" used to formulate all tablets. But they contain the same amount of the same active ingredient that Valium contains.

For the innovator companies, however, the big profit is in their brand-name products, not their generic sidelines. And the main price competition for those high-profit brands comes not from other innovator companies but from the smaller generic firms, which commonly charge the lowest prices.

Thus, brand-name firms "would have you believe that only they make that magic formula," says a senior FDA official. "But they don't. And frankly, what's required is not all that complicated."

IS THERE A DIFFERENCE IN QUALITY?

FDA inspectors visit all drug-manufacturing facilities to ensure they meet standards for equipment, workplace cleanliness, and drug quality, purity, and strength. "In most instances," says the FDA, "the generic firms have modern, state-of-the-art equipment and plants that compare favorably to or even surpass those of innovator companies."

But the real proof of generic quality resides in the drugs themselves: Do they work as well as their brand-name counterparts? Independent experts we've consulted say the answer is yes. They cite FDA approval standards as the reason.

Generic-drug approval differs from new-drug approval in one major way: Since 1984, the maker of a generic drug no longer has to carry out costly clinical trials to establish safety and efficacy for drugs introduced since 1962 by innovator companies. Such studies, says the FDA, merely redemonstrate what's already known from the original manufacturer's studies. Instead, a generic manufacturer must prove to the FDA that it has formulated the product correctly, using the same amount of the identical active ingredient as in the brand-name version.

If the generic is made properly, it will be absorbed into the bloodstream as rapidly and completely as the brand-name product it matches. The FDA test required to demonstrate this is called a bioequivalence study, a far more sophisticated procedure than the tests the agency used in earlier years for pre-1962 drugs. The generic manufacturer carries out this study on 20 to 24 healthy men. Typically, the men are first given a single dose of the generic product. Technicians take blood samples at timed intervals and then determine the amount of drug in each sample. These values are plotted over time, producing a "bioavailability curve" that describes the absorption of the drug into the bloodstream.

Later the same procedure is repeated on the same subjects, this time using the brand-name product. If the generic drug's bioavailability curve closely matches that of the brand-name drug, the FDA will approve the product. A drug that's bioequivalent to another should have the same therapeutic effect.

Bioequivalence tests enable generic companies to market their products relatively quickly and inexpensively. Rankled by that competition, the brand-name companies publicly attack the validity of the tests. Yet brand-name firms also rely on bioequivalence testing at times. Many of them reformulate their own products occasionally, adding a new coating or changing the inactive ingredients. Not surprisingly, they don't want to spend millions of dollars on clinical studies to show that the newly formulated pill also works. Instead, they do what generic firms do—carry out a bioequivalence test comparing the new formulation with the old. They then submit their data to the FDA for approval. As of 1987, Hoffmann-La Roche had gotten 13 of its formulations approved this way; American Home Products, 86; Bristol-Myers, 105.

When evaluating bioequivalence, the FDA is looking at two things: how much of the drug is absorbed into the bloodstream, and how fast. The generic must match the brand-name drug closely, but it needn't be identical. That's because two formulations of the same drug can vary slightly in their absorption and still work equally well in the body. Most pharmacological experts agree that differences of 20 percent or less are not clinically significant for most drugs. And if a generic drug differs by more than 20 percent in either the speed or amount of absorption, the FDA won't approve it.

This allowable difference is called the "plus-or-minus 20 percent rule." The brand-name companies insist that the variability allowed for generics is much too great. They've distorted the carefully established rule into a scary hypothetical situation that goes like this:

A patient takes Generic X, whose bioavailability tested as 120 percent of the brand-name's. The patient's prescription is then refilled with another version of the drug, Generic Y, whose bioavailability is 80 percent of the brand-name's. While both versions are within the plus-or-minus 20 percent rule, the change from 120 percent to 80 percent means a 33 percent decrease in bioavailability—and, it's claimed, drug therapy that may no longer be effective.

Brand-name companies call this scenario "the dangers of indiscriminate interchange." It sends a clear message to physicians: Generics may differ from each other in bioavailability. So play it safe and stick with the dependable brand-name product.

Actually, the differences among versions of a drug are extremely small. In 1986, the FDA reviewed all new generics it had approved since 1984. It calculated the average difference in bioavailability between brand-name drugs and their generic copies to be only 3.5 percent—no greater than the difference between one batch of a brand-name drug and another batch off the same assembly line. So far, about 5000 generics have been approved as bioequivalent to brand-name products. The FDA stated that it is not aware of a single documented case in which any of the 5000 generics has caused a treatment problem.

Those claiming it's dangerous to switch from one version of a drug to another are deceiving the public. The only exceptions are a few "critical" drugs that have a narrow range between blood levels that are ineffective, effective, or toxic. These drugs include digoxin (Lanoxin), levothyroxine (Synthroid, Levothroid), and warfarin (Coumadin). For this small number of drugs, blood levels should be monitored when patients switch from one formulation to another.

THE THREAT OF COMPETITION

Over the past decade, organizations that pay health-care bills—the federal government, the states, and insurance companies—have sought ways to brake the rapid rise in health-care costs. In this climate, lobbying efforts by generic companies stimulated Congress to consider legislation that would make lower-priced generic drugs more widely available. The result was a new federal law, the Drug Price Competition and Patent Term Restoration Act of 1984.

The law represented a painstaking compromise between the generic drug companies and the Pharmaceutical Manufacturers Association, the trade association that represents the innovator drug companies. The innovator companies got what they wanted: longer patent protection on new drugs. Generic companies, in turn, won the right to eventually market the same chemical under its generic name without having to prove again that the chemical works. The law quickly helped spur the introduction of generic competitors for many of the leading brands.

The increased competition promises special benefit to consumers who pay for prescription drugs completely out of their own pockets, including the majority of people 65 or older. Suppose you were a diabetic taking Diabinese, Pfizer Laboratories' brand of chlorpropamide, a drug that reduces blood-sugar levels. In 1987, a major national pharmacy chain charged $31.54 for 100 tablets of Diabinese. The same chain charged $7.59 for 100 tablets of generic chlorpropamide. If you were taking one tablet a day, the cost would be about $115 a year for Diabinese, versus about $28 for the generic version.

A Federal Trade Commission report estimated that, in 1984 alone, generic drugs saved consumers approximately $236 million. Such savings are especially important to anyone who must take drugs regularly, as older people often do. People over 65 currently constitute 12 percent of the population but consume about 30 percent of all prescription drugs.

THE PROPAGANDA WAR ON GENERICS

The contrasting photographs of spiffy brand-name manufacturers and seedy generic manufacturers sent by large drug companies to New York state legislators in 1983 was just one battle in a larger war of propaganda. With increased price competition from generic companies in sight beginning in 1983, the major pharmaceutical firms opened a campaign of disparagement, confusing and frightening physicians, pharmacists, and patients alike.

Consider the propaganda put out in 1986 by Ayerst Laboratories, a division of American Home Products, when it realized it would soon face competition from generic versions of Inderal, its brand name for propranolol, a drug used for hypertension and other disorders. Inderal rang up yearly sales of $350 million and was Ayerst's most profitable drug.

Ayerst Laboratories, like all major drug companies, employs hundreds of sales representatives, called "detail persons," who make the rounds of doctors' offices. Just before generic propranolol became available, Ayerst indoctrinated its sales force with a "sales simulation" videotape. It shows a detail person telling a physician that patients on Inderal "are high-risk patients," who "need Inderal's proven therapeutic efficacy." With a generic propranolol, the doctor is told, "there's always the chance that patient response may be compromised."

Ayerst also sent out "Dear Pharmacist" letters. They discussed a pharmacist's "potential liability" if generic propranolol were dispensed instead of Inderal and something went wrong. The letter warned of "troublesome and expensive" lawsuits that would "generate adverse publicity."

The letter was labeled false and misleading by the FDA. "It serves only to confuse and intimidate pharmacists into dispensing only Inderal . . . by suggesting unknown perils," the agency wrote in a regulatory notice it sent to Ayerst. Laws in most states protect pharmacists from incurring any increased liability when they dispense an approved generic product.

The FDA has challenged similar "Dear Pharmacist" and "Dear Doctor" letters sent by other companies, including Sandoz and A. H. Robins. The FDA regards such letters from drug firms as part of a drug's labeling; the agency can thus take action when a letter is false or misleading.

But the FDA has no authority over similar letters sent by "public interest" groups. In the summer of 1985, California pharmacists received a notice headlined "Generic Alert!!!" It was sent by Pharmacists Planning Service Inc., a nonprofit educational organization. Pharmacists were warned of lawsuits that could arise if they didn't dispense "brand-name propranolol." A short time later, that organization received a $10,000 check from Ayerst "to support the educational goals of the Pharmacists Planning Service."

Another Ayerst "educational" grant went to the Philadelphia College of Pharmacy and Science, the country's oldest pharmacy school. In exchange, the college agreed to sponsor a new organization with the avowed aim of educating professionals and the public about "the critical role research-intensive pharmaceutical firms play in preserving health care." The organization's educational thrust tended to run in a narrow groove. "Pharmaceutical research . . . is threatened by widespread consumer use of generic drugs," said its press release. Increased generic drug use, it said, "could be catastrophic." The college disbanded the organization six months after its creation because the antigeneric propaganda had become so dominant.

Ayerst nevertheless got its message across through a speakers' bureau staffed by physicians and pharmacology professors, who are paid to travel around the country on media tours. These tours resulted in over two dozen newspaper articles, with headlines such as "Warning Sounded on Generic Drugs," and "Some Doctors Still Uneasy About Generics." The articles often omit the speakers' affiliation with Ayerst.

Such antigeneric campaigns occur with "predictable regularity," according to Peter Rheinstein, M.D., director of the FDA's office of drug standards. "Every time a brand-name drug becomes vulnerable to generic competition, the makers do whatever they can to protect their market."

The campaigns seem to have an impact. Surveys show that physicians, pharmacists, and consumers prefer brand-name drugs to generics. According to a 1985 Federal Trade Commission report, when prescriptions give pharmacists a choice between dispensing a brand-name drug or its generic equivalent, they dispensed the generic only about 15 percent of the time. Their reluctance stemmed partly from fear of liability, the FTC report found. It also found that consumers tend to "equate price with quality," especially for "high perceived risk" products like drugs.

Doubts about generics make some consumers refuse them or even switch to a different pharmacy—another reason pharmacists haven't embraced generics. But as health-care cost-containment efforts continue, this cool reception to generics should gradually warm.

Advertising Rx Drugs Directly to Consumers

Traditionally, prescription drugs have been advertised only to physicians, usually through professional journals and medical trade magazines. Federal law requires such ads to carry an FDA-approved summary of the drug's side effects, contraindications, warnings, and precautions—all meant to provide prescribing physicians with balanced information about the drug.

Advertisers have no problem giving physicians balanced drug information in ads. The phrasing can be highly technical, since it's aimed at those who understand the technicalities. But consumer ads are something else again. Some summaries of risks and benefits require pages of small print, often not comprehensible to consumers.

So, in recent years, manufacturers began advertising their prescription products—without all the details—directly to the public, circumventing physicians and pharmacists alike. The practice stopped abruptly—with few exceptions—when the FDA called for a voluntary moratorium in 1983. The agency was concerned that high-pressure ad compaigns might encourage consumers to demand that their physicians prescribe inappropriate products. Most physicians, pharmacists, and consumers shared that concern.

Since then, the FDA has settled on a compromise arrangement: Ads that mention the product's name must include prescribing and precautionary information similar to that found on a package insert. This rules out radio and television commercials, but print ads can sometimes accommodate the extra information. The way around this prohibition is for the manufacturer to warn about a health problem, hint that medication is available, and urge you to see your physician or pharmacist—who will presumably dispense the mystery product. However, the FDA objects to any ad—with or without the product name—that promotes the only available treatment for a condition.

The opposition to consumer ads among medical professionals is not surprising. Ad campaigns can build powerful expectations for particular products. Patients may then be confused by a doctor's choice of some other course of treatment. Ads may also induce consumers to pressure physicians to prescribe inappropriate products. At the very least, physicians are concerned about the time they might have to spend answering ad-prompted inquiries on products that aren't appropriate for a patient's treatment.

Does anyone but drug manufacturers support the advertising of prescription drugs directly to consumers? The media that would carry the ads apparently do. In 1984, the CBS television network said that, according to a survey it had taken, consumers want more drug information—especially in such areas as safety, efficacy, and proper use. In a press release about the survey, CBS said that "health care communications can be improved through direct-to-consumer advertising of prescription drugs which meets high standards of education and information."

But nothing in the CBS survey itself indicated that consumers wanted—or would trust—advertising as a source of prescription-drug information. Indeed, an FDA report cited an independent study showing that only 9 percent of surveyed consumers considered advertising an appropriate way to disseminate information about prescription drugs. More reasonable sources of drug information would be books, educational courses in schools, and package inserts written for patients—as well as consultation with a reliable physician or pharmacist. (The most comprehensive—and comprehensible—source of unbiased information on over 5000 prescription and over-the-counter drugs is *Drug Information for the Consumer,* prepared by the United States Pharmacopeial Convention and now available in a Consumer Reports Books edition.)

Manufacturers and other supporters of direct-to-consumer prescription drug ads may presume to educate the public, but no doubt they especially want to sell more drugs. Most of the ads that promoted brand-name products did so by undermining confidence in their generic equivalents. Ever resourceful, these manufacturers have had to make do with other means to achieve the same end. And that they have done.

Undermining Generics with Worrisome Tales

During a congressional hearing in April 1987, Gerald Mossinghoff, president of the Pharmaceutical Manufacturers Association, was asked if he could assure consumers that generics were as effective as brand-name drugs.

He could not. "We have trouble with the Food and Drug Administration's tests for generic drugs," said Mossinghoff. "In some cases that test, we think, is not sharply defined. It led, for example, in November to the Epilepsy Institute putting out a physicians' alert saying some anticonvulsive drugs were *not* effective. So I am not in a position, Congressman, to give you that assurance."

The Epilepsy Institute is a nonprofit organization in New York City. On November 3, 1986, the institute issued a three-page medical-alert bulletin, headlined "GENERIC MEDICATIONS LINKED TO RENEWED SEIZURE ACTIVITY IN PEOPLE WITH EPILEPSY." The text warned against generic versions of three brand-name drugs: Tegretol, Dilantin, and Depakene, made by Ciba-Geigy, Warner-Lambert, and Abbott, respectively. The warning went to 7000 physicians and to some 100 media outlets.

The Epilepsy Institute's bulletin has been cited many times as proof that generic drugs can endanger health.

Boston's CBS television affiliate broadcast a segment, seen by 300,000 people, that began, "Well, the health of nearly five million people with seizure disorders might be in jeopardy now because of a generic drug that's been approved by the FDA." Articles conveying the warning appeared in *Medical World News, Woman's Day,* the *Boston Globe,* the *Arizona Republic,* and other publications.

Four months earlier the Epilepsy Institute's president, Ira Brody, had written a letter soliciting money from three drug companies: Ciba-Geigy, Warner-Lambert, and Abbott. In his letter, Brody listed various institute "programs" that needed financial support: educational pamphlets for drugstores, seminars for physicians, and the institute's *New York Journal of Epilepsy,* which needed advertising so that it could appear quarterly.

Brody scored with all three firms. Ciba-Geigy agreed to pay $4000 for a five-page ad in the spring 1987 issue of the journal. Warner-Lambert agreed to advertise in the summer 1987 issue. Abbott would sponsor the fall 1987 issue and would also donate $22,000 for brochures and another $8000 to sponsor a seminar. Brody said there was "no connection whatsoever" between their contributions and the decision to issue the medical-alert bulletin. "It's just doing good fundraising," he said. "We solicit funds from companies that have a vested interest in us."

The Epilepsy Institute decided to sound the alarm, its bulletin said, "after receiving and confirming scores of reports" showing that seizure-free epileptics had convulsions after being "switched from brand-name pharmaceuticals to generics."

When asked about the "scores of reports," Brody called it a "typist's exaggeration," saying the actual number of cases was 23. The institute "confirmed" eight of those, he said.

The bulletin quoted Hart deC. Peterson, M.D., professor of neurology and pediatrics at New York Hospital–Cornell Medical Center and former chairman of the Epilepsy Institute's professional advisory board. The FDA contacted Peterson. In a November 1986 letter, the agency asked him for "all available data that you have on these alleged therapeutic failures." It offered to send an investigator to look at records. Peterson did not accept the offer.

In 1987, CU contacted Peterson about the reports. "They're hearsay," he said. "But the inclination is to believe at least some of it. If I could get any good solid cases and I could prove them, I certainly would. I personally haven't seen any really good cases where switching to a generic has caused problems."

Meanwhile, foes of generic drugs were having a field day with the Epilepsy Institute's bulletin. Ciba-Geigy, maker of Tegretol, paid eight New York neurologists $100 each to attend a dinner discussion of their product. While the restaurant served pasta, Ciba-Geigy served up the Epilepsy Institute's medical-alert bulletin.

"It made us feel anxious about switching our patients to a generic drug," said a physician who was present. "After all, this reputable institution had issued an alert."

The Medical Tribune, a medical-news tabloid that is mailed free to more than 100,000 physicians, gave the story page-one treatment. The paper, which has long crusaded against generic drugs, was published by Arthur Sackler, M.D., who died in 1987. Sackler had concurrently owned an advertising agency that served many innovator drug firms.

Louis Lasagna, M.D., dean of Tufts University's Sackler School of Graduate Biomedical Studies and one of the nation's most outspoken opponents of generic drugs, also stressed the epilepsy theme in a debate presented in *USA Today.* "Doctors," he said, "hear stories, like those from the Epilepsy Institute, and are justifiably concerned. It only takes a few cases to engender anxiety."

That, of course, is exactly the purpose of such anecdotal scare tactics.

Another nonprofit organization has also fronted for a major drug company in spreading fear of generics. In December 1986, local news shows on 23 television stations ran a chilling two-minute segment that featured an 11-year-old girl clutching her throat as she demonstrated what happened when she was switched from her brand-name asthma medication to a generic version. "It's like someone strangling you," said the girl. "And it hurts, and you can't get enough air through."

The reporter concluded with this advice: "If you take medication for a chronic illness—diabetes, asthma, epilepsy, or heart disease—you should ask your physician to indicate—*in writing*—'Dispense As Written' or 'Do Not Substitute' on your next prescription."

The story, seen by an estimated 1.3 million people, was actually a "video news release"—a commercial message masquerading as news. The sponsor of this commercial message was listed as the "Asthma and Allergy Foundation of America, Los Angeles Chapter." But its $30,000 cost was paid by Key Pharmaceuticals. Key (now part of Schering-Plough Corp.) makes *Theo-Dur,* a drug for asthma. *Theo-Dur* had lost 20 percent of its $100-million-a-year market to theophylline, the generic product vilified in the commercial.

Schering-Plough claims that the commercial message was an "important public service announcement." But the Asthma and Allergy Foundation feels differently. "The Los Angeles chapter saw it as an opportunity to get some publicity," said David Branson, president of the national foundation. "But it was a mistake. They shouldn't have done it."

CU spoke with one of the asthmatic girl's physicians. He reported that her physicians made no effort to confirm that the generic drug was actually the cause of her breathing problem.

The FDA has followed up on these publicized reports of "bad" generics. According to FDA's Rheinstein, the result is always the same: "You ask for documentation and you get evasion." Yet such reports proliferate. FDA officials say that these anecdotes are a key part of the antigeneric campaign. By having a nonprofit organization spread the word, the drug company avoids FDA charges of deceptive advertising.

Campaigning for Medical Hearts and Minds

Promotional efforts, whether deceptive or not, are the lifeblood of the prescription-drug business. Major drug companies generally spend more each year on promotion than on research. Most of that promotion money is lavished on physicians—and it has an impact.

"Most doctors are brainwashed," the director of medicine at a hospital in Westchester County, New York, told CU. "I know some very intelligent practitioners who always prescribe brand-name medications and would never think of prescribing a generic product."

Years ago, physicians had some cause to be wary of generic drugs. In 1969, millions of capsules of ineffective tetracycline were recalled. In 1971, problems were reported involving one generic version of digoxin. Now, however, the FDA's more rigorous generic approval process makes such failures extremely unlikely.

Isolated cases of illegal generics have also influenced physicians' perceptions. In 1979, the FDA found that three firms were illegally marketing unapproved and ineffective versions of furosemide, a diuretic. Many doctors still refuse to prescribe generic furosemide, turning instead to the more expensive brand-name drug, Lasix.

Such problems with low-quality or illegal generics have been extremely rare. But physicians remember those incidents. And brand-name drug companies try to make sure they never forget.

The effort to influence physicians starts while they are still in training. To familiarize interns and residents with their brands, companies practically give drugs away to hospital pharmacies. The practicing physician encounters drug-company influence everywhere. Drug companies sponsor seminars, conferences, breakfasts, luncheons, dinners, and awards. They give away books, slides, and video- and audiotapes. They entertain lavishly at medical conventions. (For a meeting of the American Academy of Family Physicians, SmithKline Beckman rented Disneyland for an evening to entertain physicians and their families.)

A major part of a drug company's promotional budget goes to two areas: advertising in medical journals and fielding a marketing sales force. In leafing through the journals, a physician will encounter thousands of ads each year. They rarely mention drug prices. As a result, most physicians know very little about the cost of the medicines they prescribe. Drug company sales representatives provide physicians with much of the information they receive about drugs. They also give doctors free drug samples as well as pens, note pads, prescription pads, calendars, and other merchandise.

But increasingly, sales reps influence physicians in other ways. Ciba-Geigy, for example, has placed special emphasis on "Peer Influence" programs designed to get physicians to influence other physicians. One such program involves clinical conferences. A sales rep gets a group of physicians together for lunch or dinner. They're shown a videotaped case history and then asked for their ideas on possible therapy. The idea, a sales rep says, is to include at least one or two physicians who use the Ciba-Geigy product. That way, "they can tell success stories of their therapy that may rub off" on the other physicians.

Then there are the seminars in paradise. Large firms regularly send the nation's most influential specialists and their spouses on all-expenses-paid trips to tropical climes. In 1986, for instance, Ciba-Geigy flew 100 gynecologists to Cancún, Mexico, to bone up on Estraderm, the company's new estrogen skin patch.

Generating Sales Income to Fund More "Research"

In 1985, the top 50 pharmaceutical companies officially spent $1.26 billion on "promotion," according to industry sources. But the total amount spent to influence physicians is actually far greater. According to FDA sources, drug companies often charge costly promotional activities, such as convention entertaining and the far-flung seminars, to their education or research budgets. The FDA sources estimated in 1987 that total promotional spending by major drug companies exceeds $4 billion a year, or almost $9000 per doctor.

Many physicians prescribe brand-name drugs specifically to reward the innovator companies that develop new drugs. They figure the company will use the sales income on research that will lead to better drugs in the future. Innovator companies naturally encourage this attitude among doctors. They warn that increased sales of generics will cut into their profits and prevent them from investing in the necessary research.

But a congressional study suggests that research doesn't get top priority. In 1987, the House subcommittee on health and the environment investigated recent hikes in prescription-drug prices—a 12.2 percent increase between July 1985 and April 1987 (versus only a 2.7 percent increase in the Consumer Price Index during that time). The subcommittee staff obtained revenue data from the nation's 25 largest drug companies and prepared a report. Subcommittee chairman Henry Waxman summarized the findings at a hearing:

"Most of the money generated by the recent enormous price increases is *not* going to fund R&D [research and development]. Between the years 1982 and 1986, drug-price increases produced revenue gains of $4.7 billion. During the same period, R&D expenditures rose only $1.6 billion— or about a third of the revenue gains from price increases."

The antigeneric campaign numbers many consumers among its casualties. Some are patients who pay brand-name prices for medication available at a fraction of the cost. But the casualties also include taxpayers.

Medicaid pays the prescription bills of many low-income people—and those costs are shared by the federal government and the states. The New Jersey Health Department analyzed the cost of 2.6 million Medicaid prescriptions the state had paid for in 1985. All of the drugs were available in both brand-name and generic form. Each brand-name prescription cost the state an average of $12.39; the average generic prescription cost $6.66.

RECOMMENDATIONS

To realize the savings offered by generic drugs, you need the cooperation of both your physician and your pharmacist.

Physicians usually write the brand name when they prescribe drugs. It's shorter and easier to remember than the generic name. And since the brand name had no generic competition during the long life of its patent, the doctor is probably accustomed to writing it.

That medical habit doesn't prevent you from buying generically. The laws in all 50 states allow pharmacists to substitute a less-expensive generic version when the physician prescribes by brand. Indeed, the physician must make a conscious effort to *limit* the pharmacist to the brand name. In some states, that means he or she must write out "dispense as written" or some other phrase. In other states, the physician signs on one of two lines on the prescription pad if the pharmacist must dispense the brand specified, or signs on the other line if a generic may be substituted.

The major drug companies lobby fiercely for two-line prescription pads. Physicians seldom bother to write out "dispense as written"; but studies show that when doctors must merely choose one of the two lines, they sign the brand-name line more than half the time. Some drug companies try to make the choice for both patient and physician. They give doctors preprinted prescription pads with the brand name and the words "dispense as written," in the doctor's handwriting, on each form. This "professional courtesy" sticks you with the brand-name drug and its premium price. It's also illegal in several states.

Your physician, therefore, may represent a hurdle to your getting a generic drug. You must explicitly ask your physician to write the prescription so that it permits a generic version to be dispensed.

What if your physician doesn't know whether a generic version of the drug you need is yet available? That doesn't matter; the pharmacist will know. Whether the pharmacist will dispense the generic is a different question. Drug-company propaganda has led many pharmacists to fear that dispensing generic drugs may result in lawsuits.

So once again, you must take the initiative. Tell your pharmacist that you want the least expensive version of the drug that's been prescribed for you. Usually, that will be the generic version. Occasionally, the brand-name version may be cheaper—if the pharmacist has gotten a special deal from the maker, for example.

Drug prices vary widely from pharmacy to pharmacy. So shop around, checking both chain stores and independent pharmacies. Many pharmacies now give out price information over the phone.

If you switch from a brand name to a generic, don't worry if its color and shape are different from the brand-name product you've been taking. (Brand-name makers may sue generic firms whose products duplicate the appearance of brand-name drugs.) The product's appearance won't affect how the drug works.

GLOSSARY

This list of medical terms is selected primarily from the pages of *The New Medicine Show.* Words and phrases defined here include those occurring in more than one chapter, those indispensable to understanding the material in a chapter, and those that may help clarify some of the definitions themselves. This last criterion is reflected in the frequent use of **bold face** as a guide to other terms in the glossary.

Not listed in the glossary are the names of drugs (over-the-counter and prescription), the names of most diseases, and words adequately defined in the book. Although the definitions can ease reading of *The New Medicine Show,* they should also be of help in understanding other references to medical matters.

Absorption A process by which **drugs** and foods pass through a barrier, such as the intestinal wall or the skin, into the bloodstream.

Acid A broad category of chemical substances, marked among other things by sour taste and a propensity to react with **alkaline** substances (bases) to form salts. Most bodily functions depend upon the maintenance of a balance between acids and bases in cells, blood, and other body fluids. (See also **acidification, buffered, neutralizing capacity.**)

Acidification (urinary) In a healthy body, **acids** and bases are kept in balance by the excretion of acid in the urine. Certain **drugs** such as ascorbic acid (vitamin C) may increase the concentration of acid in the urine. The ability of the kidneys to excrete acid is impaired by certain diseases.

Acute Describing an illness that comes on suddenly with strong sharp **symptoms** (such illnesses are usually of short duration), or any disease that needs urgent medical attention. (See also **chronic.**)

Addicting, Addiction Describing the property of certain **drugs,** such as alcohol, **barbiturates,** and **narcotics,** that leads to compulsive use by some people. Addiction generally manifests itself in three ways: **Tolerance** to the drug develops so that the user no longer obtains the effect achieved with earlier dosage; physical withdrawal **symptoms,** sometimes even life-threatening, occur for a time if use of the addicting drug is curtailed; and recurrent craving for the drug is experienced even long after recovery from withdrawal symptoms.

Administration The method of introducing a **drug** into a patient's body. It includes dosage (how much), schedule (how often), and route (by mouth, by injection, etc.). (See also **regimen, systemic, topical.**)

Adrenal Glands A pair of **endocrine** glands, one perched atop each kidney.

Among the major products of the adrenal glands' outer or **cortical** layer are the **corticosteroids,** notably **cortisone** and hydrocortisone. The inner core or medulla produces **adrenaline.**

Adrenaline A **hormone** secreted by the inner core or medulla of the **adrenal glands.** It acts on diverse organs and systems of the body to prepare one for "fight or flight," or other stressful situations. It is also available as the drug epinephrine (Adrenalin).

Adsorb See **bind.**

Alkali, Alkaline The chemical opposite of **acid.** Synonym: base. When an alkaline substance reacts with an **acid,** the two **neutralize** each other and form a salt. Lye is a common alkaline substance. (See also **acidification, buffered, neutralizing capacity.**)

Allergen A substance (usually a protein) that causes an **allergy.**

Allergy A person's abnormal reaction to a substance called an **allergen.** It results from the body's immune mechanism being overwhelmed. **Symptoms** may include runny nose, red and itchy eyes, skin rash, wheezing, or sneezing. These symptoms are usually caused by the release of histamine. (See also **antihistamine, desensitization.**)

Amino Acids Basic chemical units into which food proteins are broken down during digestion, and from which body proteins are built up in various cells and organs, such as the liver.

Analgesic A **drug,** such as aspirin or codeine, that decreases pain.

Analogue A chemical **compound** similar in structure to another chemical compound and having the same effect on body processes.

Anaphylactic, Anaphylaxis An **acute** allergic response—manifested by cardiovascular collapse—to an **allergen** to which a person has been previously sensitized. Anaphylactic shock can be fatal.

Anatomic Having to do with the shape, structure, and relative position of the body's various parts, as distinct from their function (physiology) or malfunction (pathology).

Anemia A reduction in the number of red blood cells whose function it is to distribute oxygen to all parts of the body. Anemic blood looks "washed out"—and that's the way to describe how the patient feels.

Anesthetic A **drug** used to deaden pain or to cause loss of consciousness. A local anesthetic dulls sensation at a specific spot or over a small portion of the body; a general anesthetic banishes pain by bringing on a deep artificial sleep; a **topical** anesthetic works only on the area of skin to which it is applied.

Anorexia A **pathological** loss of appetite; aversion to food.

Antacid Short for antiacid—an **alkaline compound** that **neutralizes acid,** especially in the stomach.

Antibiotic A substance that can kill harmful **microorganisms** in the body, or else keep them from multiplying until the body's own defenses can destroy them. Broad-spectrum antibiotics attack a wide range of germs; narrow-spectrum ones zero in on specific types. Unlike **antiseptics,** antibiotics can be made by living organisms—**fungi**—from which they are extracted and refined for **pharmacological** use. They can also be synthesized in the laboratory.

Antibody A protein substance made by certain **white blood** cells in the body in response to injection, **ingestion,** or inhalation of an **antigen.** The production of an antibody can be beneficial, as in the case of immunization. (See also **immunological response, vaccine.**)

Anticoagulant A **drug** used to retard the clotting of blood. Typical anticoagulants are heparin (Meparin, Panheprin) and warfarin (Athrombin-K, Coumadin, Panwarfin).

Antigen A substance that causes the body's immune system to make a specific **antibody** that will react with (or **neutralize**) that antigen. (See also **immunological response, vaccine.**)

Antihistamine A **drug** used to treat an **allergy** by counteracting the effects of histamine, a chemical manufactured by certain cells in the body.

Antihypertensive A drug taken by a person with **hypertension** to lower blood pressure and keep it lowered.

Antipruritic A medication used to relieve itching. There are **topical** antipruritics, such as calamine lotion; others are taken by mouth.

Antipyretic A **drug,** such as aspirin or acetaminophen, that lowers fever.

Antiseptic A chemical substance that prevents **infection** by destroying **microorganisms** on the skin, or curtails their multiplication. (See also **antibiotic, germicidal.**)

Assay To analyze and quantify a substance.

Astringent A substance that makes blood vessels or other tissues "pucker up" or contract. Alum, the material in styptic pencils, is a typical astringent used to stop small cuts from bleeding.

Asymptomatic Without **symptoms;** signifying that an **infection** or disease is in a latent stage, is in **remission,** or simply is cured.

Atonic Flaccid, lacking **tone.** When a nerve is injured, the muscle supplied by that nerve becomes atonic. When intestinal muscles are atonic, **peristalsis** is inadequate and the result is almost always constipation.

Atrophy A decrease in size and function of a part of the body from lack of use or from disruption of nerve supply, blood flow, or **hormone** delivery to that part of the body.

Bacteria General name for a vast variety of **microorganisms,** including beneficial as well as harmful types. "Good" bacteria make yogurt, aid digestion, and help nourish growing plants. "Bad" or disease-producing bacteria cause all manner of infectious diseases.

Bacterial Resistance   When a person acquires **immunity** against a strain of **bacteria,** that's good. But when the bacteria develop immunity of their own against an **antibiotic,** that's resistance—and that's bad.

Barbiturate   A type of **drug** used in small doses as a **sedative,** and in larger doses as a **hypnotic.** Barbiturates can be **addicting.**

Belladonna Alkaloids   A mixture of plant derivatives including atropine, scopolamine, and related chemicals. As a group, the belladonna alkaloids work against the **parasympathetic nervous system.** One of their actions is to dry **secretions** of the **mucous membranes** in the mouth, nose, and stomach.

Bind (Adsorb)   To enter into a chemical bond, as when one substance unites or combines firmly with another.

Biochemical   Having to do with the chemical composition of the body as well as its **metabolism,** rather than its anatomy or physiology.

Biopsy   Surgical removal of a small slice or sliver of tissue for examination, usually under a microscope, to see if its cells are cancerous or otherwise abnormal.

Blind Trial   A **controlled trial** of a **drug** in which the patients do not know whether they are being given the real thing or a **placebo**—but their doctors know. (See also **double-blind trial.**)

Bone Marrow Failure   Marrow, the soft pith or filling inside bones, manufactures the blood's red cells (which deliver oxygen throughout the body), **white cells** (which fight **infection**), and platelets (which help **clotting**). Certain **drugs,** as well as radiation, damage marrow so it cannot produce these cells; the phenomenon that results is bone marrow failure. Bone marrow failure may be partial, affecting only one type of blood cell rather than all three.

Bronchi   Plural of bronchus; subdivisions of the trachea (windpipe), which further subdivide into bronchioles (narrower and narrower air tubes) descending deep into the lungs. Bronchitis is the name for **inflammation** of the bronchi.

Buffered   Describing therapeutic preparations to which **antacids** have been added. In the case of aspirin, buffering supposedly protects the stomach against the corrosive effect of the aspirin.

Capillary   The very finest subdivision of the body's network of blood vessels, the capillary is a microscopic blood vessel, much finer than a hair, with ultra-thin walls, through which the blood gives up its oxygen to the body's tissues.

Carcinogenic   Cancer-causing. (See also **mutagenic.**)

Carrier   In **drugs** and cosmetics, the (relatively) **inert** substance in which the active ingredient is dissolved, mixed, or suspended for ease of **administration.**

Central Nervous System   The brain and spinal cord together serve as a command module that governs branching networks of peripheral nerves and the

sympathetic nervous system. The central nervous system also controls thinking, dreaming, and consciousness.

Chemical Cauterization A burning away of unwanted living tissue (warts, for example) by means of caustic **compounds,** such as strong **acids** or **alkalies.**

Chemotherapy Treatment of disease **(therapy)** by medicating with chemical **compounds.** Synonym: **drug** therapy.

Chromosomes The thousands of genes that carry hereditary messages from parents to offspring are strung on forty-six microscopic "necklaces" called chromosomes. The chromosomes are tightly coiled inside most body cells, including sperm and ova. These strings of **genetic** beads can be broken and partly lost or wrongly restrung by certain chemicals, infectious agents, radiation, and other factors—thus causing birth defects.

Chronic Describing a disease of long duration or one that is recurrent. (See also **acute.**)

Clinical Having to do with the medical care of ill people, and treatment of their signs and **symptoms,** as distinct from experimentation with laboratory animals. Thus a clinical trial involves trying new **therapy** on human subjects.

Clinician A practicing physician. Besides treating sick people, the clinician may (or may not) teach medicine and take part in medical research.

Clotting Mechanism The body's self-sealing system. When blood is shed, a complex series of **biochemical** reactions starts. The process ends with the manufacture of a tough substance called fibrin, which closes the wound and stops the bleeding. Certain **anticoagulants,** such as heparin (Meparin, Panheprin) and warfarin (Athrombim-K, Coumadin, Panwarfin), can disrupt this clotting or **coagulation** mechanism. Aspirin is also an anticlotting agent by dint of its effects on platelets. The clotting mechanism is defective in people afflicted with clotting factor deficiencies such as hemophilia.

Coagulation What happens to the white of an egg when it's boiled. A complex **biochemical** process by which the blood forms solid clumps or clots to staunch a bleeding wound and thus start the healing process. (See also **thrombosed.**)

Compound In medical parlance, a preparation formed by combining several ingredients according to a formula. In chemical terms, a uniform substance formed by the stable combination of two or more chemical elements, as distinct from a mere mixture. (See also **molecular structure.**)

Congenital Present at birth and usually arising during the **fetus's** development in the uterus. Congenital defects or malformations are either **genetic**—inherited from one or both parents—or produced during pregnancy (as by a **drug** the woman may have used) or resulting from a **virus** or other **infection** the pregnant woman may have acquired and passed on to the **embryo** or fetus.

Congestion The disruption of function in certain parts of the body by swelling of the lining tissues and by partial obliteration of the normal channels of blood flow or air flow. For instance, in **congestive heart failure,** congestion of the lungs occurs, making breathing arduous. Nasal congestion means swelling of the **mucous membranes** of the nose, making breathing through the nose difficult.

Congestive Heart Failure A disorder characterized by swelling of the ankles and by shortness of breath. Congestive heart failure may follow a heart attack when the heart muscle has been severely damaged and thus can no longer function efficiently as a pump. Heart failure may also result from other forms of heart disease or from lung disease. (See also **coronary heart disease.**)

Connective Tissue The "cement" of the body in which most cells are embedded. Connective tissue is made up for the most part of a material called collagen. Certain diseases, such as rheumatoid arthritis (see **rheumatology**), rheumatic fever, and lupus erythematosus, are disorders that primarily affect collagen.

Contraindication A reason not to use a given medication in a given situation; for example, many ordinarily beneficial **drugs** are contraindicated during pregnancy.

Controlled Substances Within the context of this book, certain **prescription drugs,** such as **analgesics,** that are **addicting** and for which physicians and druggists must record and report every prescription in order to prevent illicit traffic and abuse.

Controlled Trial or Study When a **drug** or other form of **therapy** is tried out **clinically,** to determine its efficacy, **toxicity, side effects,** indications, and **contraindications,** variable factors that could distort these results must be minimized. This is done by comparing the response of a trial group (patients who receive the new treatment) with that of a group of control subjects (patients who do not). The trial group and the control group are carefully matched for similarity in age, gender, and other relevant factors. (See also **blind trial, double-blind trial.**)

Coronary Heart Disease The name for the disorder that results from reduction in blood flow to the heart muscle due to narrowing of the coronary arteries by accumulation of fatty substances in the walls of the arteries. Activities that increase the heart rate can then cause transient chest pains (known as angina pectoris). If a narrowed coronary artery becomes completely blocked by a blood clot (coronary thrombosis), the portion of the heart muscle supplied by that artery usually ceases to function. This is known as a heart attack—technically, myocardial infarction. (See also **congestive heart failure.**)

Corrosive Capable of destroying tissue, as a strong **acid** or **alkali.**

Cortical Referring to the outer layer of certain organs. For instance, the cortical layer of the **adrenal glands** (adrenal cortex) secretes **cortico-steroids.**

Corticosteroid A family of potent, versatile **hormones** originating mainly in the **adrenal glands,** used therapeutically to treat **inflammatory** and allergic diseases. A corticosteroid can be produced naturally in the adrenal glands or synthesized in the laboratory.

Cortisone A **corticosteroid** that can be made in the body or synthesized in the laboratory. Introduced in 1952, this chemical is useful in treating many diseases but may have serious long-term **side effects.**

Culture A method of growing cells or **microorganisms** in the laboratory in order to identify them and to determine their resistance to **antibiotics.** The special food on which they are grown is the culture **medium.** (See also **in vitro, in vivo.**)

Cyclic Repeating on a regular periodic on-again, off-again schedule.

Decongestant A substance—usually a **vasoconstrictor**—that relieves nasal **congestion.**

Degenerative Referring to changes in bodily function that reflect deterioration of certain cells or tissues, and the substances they secrete. For example, osteoarthritis is a degenerative joint disease.

Dehydration Loss of water from the body or any of its tissues, beyond normal sweating and urination. If mild, it triggers thirst to restore the fluid balance; if severe and sudden (for example, as a result of massive diarrhea), dehydration can cause shock and death, especially in young children.

Demulcent A substance that soothes, softens, or protects a **mucous membrane** surface. An **emollient** does the same for skin.

Dependence Can be physical or psychological. Physical dependence is synonymous with **addiction.** Psychological dependence may be equated with the **placebo** effect.

Depressant A **drug,** such as a **barbiturate** or alcohol, that acts on the **central nervous system** to diminish mental acuity and muscular activity.

Dermatitis An **inflammation** of the skin due to any of many causes, known and unknown. Thus, contact dermatitis is a rash occurring as a reaction to some irritating chemical, textile, or other material touching or rubbing the skin. (See also **eczema.**)

Desensitization A process by which **allergy** is reduced by periodic injection of gradually increasing amounts of the offending **allergen.** A more accurate term for this process is hyposensitization because complete desensitization is rarely achieved.

Detoxify To remove or neutralize the harmful activity of a **toxic** substance in the body.

Diabetes Mellitus An all-too-familiar disorder of **metabolism,** in which the body cannot assimilate sugar for lack—or relative lack—of the pancreatic **hormone** insulin. Popularly shortened to diabetes.

Diathermy   Deep heat **therapy,** generated by microwaves, aimed at muscles and joints. A microwave oven uses a similar principle.

Digitally   Refers to an examination technique in which the physician uses a finger (as in a rectal examination).

Diuretic   A **drug** that acts to eliminate fluid from the body by increasing the amount of urine released.

Double-Blind Trial   A **controlled trial** of a **drug** in a **clinical** situation in which neither the recipients nor the experimenters (hence: double) know which patients are receiving the active substance, and which are being given a **placebo.** This dual ignorance minimizes subjective reactions to the drug being tested. (See also **blind trial.**)

Drug   Medical meaning: Any chemical agent or medicinal substance (**compound,** preparation, remedy, etc.) used to promote health or to treat disease by causing a desired change within the body or on its surface. Popular meaning: Certain chemical compounds and plant substances that alter mood or mental or emotional state; some of these drugs are **addicting.**

Duodenal Ulcer   When the highly **acid** gastric juices of the stomach eat away at the wall of the duodenum (the first part of the small intestine below the stomach), the resulting raw sore is a duodenal ulcer. A duodenal ulcer can be painful and can bleed. If the ulcer heals with excessive scar tissue, an intestinal obstruction may result. (See also **peptic ulcer.**)

Eczema   A type of **dermatitis,** usually caused by an **allergy.**

Electroencephalographic   Relating to the electroencephalograph (EEG)—a machine that helps a neurologist diagnose brain **tumors,** epilepsy, and other disorders by detecting abnormalities in the electrical waves emanating from different areas of the brain. Similar to the electrocardiograph (ECG)—a machine that helps a physician detect electrical impulses from the heart.

Elixir   A liquid form of the sugar-coated pill. A mixture of water, sweetener, scent, and alcohol, used as a **carrier** to make medicine pleasant tasting.

Embryo   The earliest stage of human develop in the uterus from the time the ovum has been fertilized until about two months later. (See also **fetus.**)

Emetic   A substance that provokes vomiting when swallowed.

Emollient   A substance—such as petrolatum or olive oil—that soothes, softens, or protects the skin surface. A **demulcent** does the same for **mucous membrane.**

Endocrine System   An interlocking directorate of glands whose **hormones** control bodily growth, sex characteristics, **metabolism,** and many other functions. The main endocrine glands are the **adrenals,** ovaries, pancreas, parathyroids, **pituitary,** testes, and thyroid.

Entity   A specifically defined thing, usually said of a particular **molecular structure** or a characteristic disease.

Enzymes   Proteins made by the body that act as catalysts for many **biochemical** reactions. Enzymes also break down food and other substances into simpler chemical **compounds** that can then be absorbed, metabolized, or otherwise used by the body. Enzymes are also used commercially; meat tenderizer, for instance, is an enzyme.

Expectorating, Expectoration, Expectorant Coughing up and spitting out of phlegm (see also **exudate**) from the lungs and **bronchi.** An expectorant is a substance intended to ease coughing and make the **sputum** less thick.

Exudate (Pus) A thick fluid containing dead **white blood cells, microorganisms,** and solid cellular debris that oozes or leaks from the blood into tissues at the site of an **infection.**

Fetus The product of conception after graduating from its first two months of life as an **embryo** and until it becomes an infant at birth.

Folic Acid A nutrient used by the **bone marrow** in the production of red blood cells.

Free Fatty Acid An organic **acid** "freed" from a more complex **compound** (triglyceride) in the **metabolism** of body fat.

Functional Disease A disorder due to the faulty working of one or more structurally healthy organs or parts of the body. As opposed to **organic disease.**

Fungus A parasitic **microorganism,** best known as the itchy villain in athlete's foot. The category also includes some medically more important types that infect internal organs and can even cause death. Some fungi, though, are beneficial—such as the molds that produce **antibiotics,** and the yeast that makes bread rise.

Gastrointestinal Having to do with the digestive tract including the esophagus, stomach, small intestine, large intestine, and rectum. Abbreviated "GI" (as in GI series, which is an X-ray visualization of the upper part of the gastrointestinal tract taken after the patient swallows a radiopaque substance, such as barium).

Gel A substance of jellylike consistency.

Generic Describing the name given to a **drug** by the United States Adopted Names Council, as distinct from the registered brand name that a pharmaceutical company gives to its version of the same chemical preparation.

Genetic Inherited through the parents' genes. Genetic traits (such as color of hair and eyes), as well as genetic diseases and defects, run in families in more or less predictable patterns. A child inherits traits and characteristics, as well as defects or susceptibility to certain diseases. Such genetic effects may not be readily noticeable in the parents; they are passed on by union of the parental ovum and sperm, rather than by what happens during pregnancy.

Genitourinary Genital plus urinary equal genitourinary. The body's reproduction and urinary system, extending from kidneys to ureters, bladder, and **urethra** (that is, the urinary tract), plus the adjacent genital tract. In males, the latter runs from testes to prostate and penis; in females, from ovaries, Fallopian tubes, and uterus to cervix and vagina.

Germicidal Referring to chemical agents—lethal to germs—which are generally used on inanimate objects (e.g., germicidal solutions for sterilizing surgical instruments). Describes the action of certain **antiseptics.** (See also **microorganisms.**)

Glaucoma A serious eye disease caused by buildup of fluid pressure inside the eyeball. Part of the **degenerative** aging process, simple or **chronic** glaucoma usually comes on gradually; if untreated, it usually destroys the optic nerve, causing blindness. Closed-angle (also known as narrow-angle) or **acute** glaucoma has a sudden severe onset due to a narrowing of the eyeball's natural drainage channels. Acute glaucoma is accompanied by severe pain. If untreated, acute glaucoma can lead to irreparable damage.

Gluten A protein in wheat and other grains that is thought to produce a special **allergy** in susceptible people, with unpleasant digestive effects including cramps and diarrhea. A gluten-free diet is helpful in celiac disease and nontropical sprue.

Grain The apothecary's traditional unit of weight—approximately $65/1000$ of a **gram.** It is still used by doctors in prescribing—and by pharmacists in compounding—pills, powders, and potions. (See also **milligram.**)

Gram A unit of weight in the metric system, often used to measure **drugs.** Approximately 28 grams equal 1 ounce; $1/1000$ of a gram is a **milligram.** (See also **grain.**)

Gram-Negative and -Positive Bacteria are of two varieties: Gram-positive bacteria are visible under the microscope when dyed by a certain technique—Gram's stain; Gram-negative bacteria fail to hold the color. (Named after Hans Gram, a Danish bacteriologist, not after the **gram** unit of weight.)

Hallucinogen A **drug** that may cause some individuals to see or hear things that aren't real.

Halogens A group of related chemical elements—chlorine, iodine, bromine, and fluorine. They combine readily with hydrogen to form **acids,** and with metals to form salts.

Hemolytic Referring to the process of hemolysis by which the membrane surrounding a red blood cell breaks. Hemolysis may be caused by a defect in the red cell membrane itself (as in sickle cell **anemia**) or by an **antibody** that clings to and damages the red cell membrane.

Hemorrhage Excessive loss of blood from the body or into its inner cavities through cut or torn veins, arteries, or **capillaries.**

Hormone A chemical substance made in an **endocrine** gland and secreted into the bloodstream. The hormone then acts on some distant target within the body.

Host (1) An organism (especially a human being) in and on which an invading **microorganism** thrives. (2) An individual who receives a donor transplant organ.

House Staff Medical doctors enrolled in a hospital training program; popularly referred to as interns and residents.

Hyper- A prefix meaning more than normal.

Hypertension A disorder that is characterized by increased blood pressure. If undetected or untreated, hypertension may eventually affect the functioning of the brain, eyes, heart, and kidneys.

Hypnotic A **drug** that induces sleep. Some hypnotics, in smaller dosage, are used as **sedatives.**

Hypo- A prefix meaning less than normal.

Idiopathic A medical term used to describe a disease of unknown cause or origin.

Immune Mechanism See **immunological response.**

Immunity Resistance to a specific **infection.** (See also **vaccine.**)

Immunological Response The production of specific proteins called **antibodies** by certain **white blood cells** in response to stimulation by specific **antigens** (e.g., **bacteria, viruses,** pollens). The antibodies resist in varying degrees invasion of the body by these **microorganisms** and other alien substances. Transfused blood of the wrong type or an organ transplanted from another body can also induce this response.

Incidence In general, the frequency with which something happens. In particular, the rate at which disease or death occurs in a population; it is usually expressed as so many per hundred thousand individuals. Prevalence, on the other hand, is the total number of cases in an entire population. (See also **mortality.**)

Incubate To facilitate growth or multiplication of cells or germs in a **culture medium** (in vitro) to the point where they can be identified, or **in vivo** to the point where they cause **symptoms.**

Inert Without physiological action or effect, as a **placebo.**

Infection (1) Invasion of the body, or one of its parts, by a harmful **microorganism.** (2) The disease thus caused by the invasion.

Inflammation The body's four-alarm response to injury or infection: (1) pain, (2) heat, (3) reddening, and (4) swelling. These local reactions signify that the body is rallying its forces to limit and repair the damage. Inflammation is thus not the same as **infection,** although the latter often triggers inflammation.

Ingested, Ingestion Swallowed, taken by mouth into the **gastrointestinal** tract. Ingestion is the most common mode of **administration** for **drugs**—pills, powders, potions, capsules, syrups, **elixirs,** etc. Other methods include injection into bloodstream, muscle or skin, infusion, inhalation, and **absorption.**

Insult   Any injury, abuse, maltreatment, or excessive stress suffered by a cell, tissue, organ—or entire body. (See also **reversible.**)

In Vitro   Literally, "in glass"—a medical or biological event that takes place, outside the human body, in the laboratory. As opposed to **in vivo.** (See also **culture, incubate.**)

In Vivo   Literally, "in life"—a medical or biological event that takes place in a living human or animal. As opposed to **in vitro.** (See also **culture, incubate.**)

Iodide   Derived from iodine, a **halogen.** Iodide-containing salts such as sodium iodide or potassium iodide. Iodide that is **ingested** in food or medication is avidly picked up by the thyroid gland where it is used for the manufacture of thyroid **hormones.** Radioactive iodide is often used to diagnose and treat certain thyroid diseases. (See also **radioactive isotope.**)

Ionizing Radiation   High-energy radiation, such as that produced by X rays, gamma rays from **radioactive isotopes,** and nuclear fallout, which penetrate deep into bodily tissue. In high enough doses, ionizing radiation precisely aimed at **tumor** cells may kill or cripple them. But at the same time, healthy cells in its path may suffer **inflammation,** death, or transformation into malignant cells.

Irreversible   A medical term for incurable. A one-way process of deterioration that may be arrested, perhaps, but never cured.

-itis   A suffix meaning **inflammation** of, as in appendicitis.

Lactating   Producing breast milk, as a mother who breast-feeds her baby.

Lesion   Any damaged site or local **pathological** condition in skin or internal tissue, caused by disease, degeneration, or injury.

Medium   What **bacteria** feed on—the special mixture of nutrients, chemical, and fluids in which and on which **cultured** cells and **microorganisms** grow in laboratories.

Membrane   See **mucous membrane.**

Metabolism   The **biochemical** processes by which food and oxygen are used by the body to provide the energy that is necessary for the proper functioning of body organs and tissues.

Metabolite   A new substance formed in the body by **metabolism** of a given **drug** or chemical. It may act quite differently from the original substance, its **precursor.**

Microorganisms   Living creatures too small to be seen with the naked eye. **Pathological** microorganisms, which cause **infections** in larger forms of life, are known colloquially as germs. They include **viruses, bacteria,** and **fungi.**

Milligram   ¹⁄₁₀₀₀ of a gram; a unit of weight in the metric system of measurement, in which **drug** dosages can be measured. (See also **grain, gram.**)

Molecular Structure   The architecture of a **compound.** By making small changes in the molecular structure of a **drug, analogues** are produced and the **pharmacological** effects of the original substance may be altered.

Morbidity   The statistical rate at which people get sick from a specific cause.

Mortality   The statistical rate at which people die of a given cause, usually expressed as so many deaths per hundred thousand people.

Mucous Membrane   The body's "inside skin"—extremely thin, soft layers of cells that line the surface of certain body tracts such as the **respiratory** tract and the **gastrointestinal** tract.

Mucus   A colorless substance secreted by the **mucous** cells of the intestines, cervix, and **respiratory** tract.

Mutagenic   Able to alter the **genetic** message by which a given cell reproduces its kind. Such a mutation of the cell may result in cancer; the mutagenic substance is then said to be **carcinogenic** as well. Or, if the mutated cells are in the reproductive system, they may cause birth defects.

Narcotic   A natural or synthetic **addicting drug** used medically to relieve pain or to produce sleep by depressing the **central nervous system.** Examples are codeine, meperidine (Demerol), and morphine.

Nephrology   A branch of medical science dealing with the kidney—its structure, functions, and diseases.

Neutral, Neutralize   Any substance that is neither **acid** nor **alkaline** is said to be neutral. When an acid meets an alkaline substance in a test tube or the stomach, for instance, they neutralize each other to form a salt.

Neutralizing Capacity   The ability of an **alkali** to offset acidity. (See also **antacid**.)

NF   Refers to a **drug** compounded according to the *National Formulary,* a semiofficial directory of drug standards and specifications, issued every five years by the American Pharmaceutical Association. (See also **USP.**)

Nodular Thyroid   A thyroid gland that has one or more lumps that can be felt through the skin of the neck. A nodular thyroid requires evaluation by a physician.

Nostrum   A "remedy" for which extravagant, scientifically unsupported therapeutic claims are often made; a **patent medicine.**

Occlusion   In general, the closing or blocking of a blood vessel or some other passageway or orifice in the body. In dentistry, the manner in which upper and lower teeth meet when the jaws shut; the "bite."

Oncology   A branch of medical science dealing with **tumors** (particularly cancers)—their origin, nature, growth, effects, and treatment.

Organic Disease   A disorder due to **anatomic** changes in a body organ that interferes with an organ's ability to do its job. As opposed to **functional disease** of a structurally intact organ. For example, rectal cancer, an organic disease, may cause constipation. Constipation triggered by a family crisis would be a functional type of bowel disorder.

Overt   Apparent to the senses; noticeable to a patient or a physician. The opposite of **asymptomatic.**

Over-the-Counter (OTC) Drug A **drug** that the Food and Drug Administration (FDA) accepts as safe for self-medication. According to the FDA, an OTC drug can be used by consumers for disorders they diagnose themselves and treat by following the directions on the label without advice from a physician. (See also **prescription drug**.)

Parasympathetic Nervous System A network of nerves that controls such involuntary, unconscious, automatic body reactions as dilatation of certain blood vessels, slowdown in heartbeat, narrowing of pupils, salivation, and increased nasal **secretion**. The **sympathetic nervous system** generally has opposite effects.

Patent Medicine An **over-the-counter** preparation whose formula is usually a trade secret, and for which unproven therapeutic benefits are often claimed; a **nostrum**.

Pathological Describing an abnormality usually caused by disease.

Peptic Ulcer A raw, sore, eroded area on the wall of the stomach or duodenum. When the wall of the stomach or duodenum is eaten all the way through, the **lesion** is called a perforation. If a blood vessel is eroded in the process, bleeding occurs—hence the familiar bleeding ulcer.

Perforation (of ulcer) See **peptic ulcer**.

Perinatal Referring to the time period from birth to approximately one month afterward.

Peripheral Nerve A nerve that transmits pain or other sensory perceptions from the skin or limbs to the **central nervous system,** and sends the brain's messages back out again to these remote—that is, peripheral—parts of the body.

Peristalsis Synchronized, sequential contractions of special muscles in the **gastrointestinal** tract that nudge and squeeze food through the esophagus and stomach to the intestine and rectum.

Pharmacological Concerning the action—therapeutic or **toxic** or both—of a **drug** on or in the body; its **absorption, metabolism,** and excretion, as well as its effect on cells, tissues, organs, and bodily function.

Photosensitivity Reaction A heightened sensitivity of the skin to the rays of the sun, caused by certain oral medications or cosmetics.

Phytates Chemical substances, salts of phytic acid, which have the capacity to combine with calcium and iron, thus impairing the body's **absorption** of these nutrients.

Pituitary An **endocrine** gland located at the base of the brain: the body's main command module. Its **hormones** direct the activities of the **adrenal glands,** ovaries, testes, and thyroid, and also govern such key processes as growth and **metabolism.**

Placebo A medically **inert** substance formulated to mimic—in color and form—an active substance; used in testing the efficacy of a **drug**. The patients in a **blind trial** (and their doctors, as well, in a **double-blind trial**) do not know who receives the active substance, or who receives the dummy one. In some **clinical** studies as many as 40 percent of the subjects respond favorably to a placebo.

Precursor   That which comes before. Refers to (1) a chemical substance that is converted to another chemical substance (thus, flurazepam is the precursor of its long-lived **metabolite**); or (2) a previously existing disorder that leads to a disease (cystic hyperplasia may be a precursor of endometrial cancer).

Prescription Drug   A **drug** available only by a doctor's prescription; too potent or dangerous or **addicting** to be sold **over the counter.**

Pressor Agents   Chemicals (usually **drugs**) that have the effect of raising blood pressure. (See also **vasomotor.**)

Propellant   A gas or liquified gas used to provide the pressure necessary to expel the contents in a self-spraying container.

Prophylactic, Prophylaxis   Preventive: tending to guard against or forestall disease by removing its cause, or denying it a chance to develop.

Prosthetic, Prosthesis   Any artificial or "bionic" device fitted to replace or reinforce a missing or faulty part of the body—for example, a dental crown or a stainless steel hip joint.

Protocol   A plan specifying the rules and regulations for conducting any scientific study. For a **clinical** trial, a protocol lays down such conditions as how many patients will be treated by what means for how long in what manner. (See also **blind trial, double-blind trial, placebo.**)

Psychosis   One of a group of serious mental or emotional disorders, notably **schizophrenia** and manic-depressive psychosis, which may impair mental functioning sufficiently to interfere with capacity to meet the ordinary demands of life.

Psychosomatic   Referring to a group of physical ailments that are known to be caused by emotional factors. These are not imagined illnesses, but conditions in which actual evidence of physical disease can be documented. For example, irritable colon syndrome, bronchial asthma, and **peptic ulcer** are usually considered psychosomatic illnesses.

Psychotherapeutic Drug   A chemical **compound** that is prescribed by a physician in the treatment of mental or emotional disorders.

Psychotherapy   The treatment of mental or emotional disorders primarily by interaction between therapist and patient, or therapist and a group of patients, or interaction among patients without a therapist. Its methods include suggestion, persuasion, hypnosis, dream analysis, free-association analysis, transference, acting out, and other similar mechanisms.

Pulmonary   Having to do with the lungs.

Pus   See **exudate.**

Radioactive Isotope   A kind of chemical element, either natural or made in a nuclear reactor, that emits energy in the form of radiation that can be detected by instruments. The isotope of a particular element can mimic its natural counterpart in body **metabolism.** As a result, certain chemical **compounds** "tagged" with the radioactive isotope can be swallowed or injected and followed through the body by a radiation detector making possible many kinds of diagnostic tests. Large doses of radioactive isotopes may be used therapeutically.

Rebound Effect An intense flare-up of **symptoms** related to the use of medication that occurs when the medication is suddenly withdrawn or its effects wear off. The rebound symptoms are generally more severe than those for which the medication was originally taken. In order to suppress these symptoms the patient may resort to more frequent use of the medication or increased dosage or both. The rebound effect most commonly occurs with the use of nose drops. It also occurs with abrupt discontinuance of **corticosteroids** and occasionally other oral medications.

Reflex An automatic, involuntary action of a muscle in response to nerve stimulation. An unconditioned reflex is one built into the nervous system of every normal human being (e.g., the knee-jerk reaction). A conditioned reflex is one that has been learned by experience (e.g., a dog drooling at the sound of a dinner bell).

Regimen Just what the doctor orders; any therapeutic program or schedule for eating, sleeping, exercising, taking medicine, and so forth.

Regurgitate To vomit; throw up.

Remission Temporary absence of signs and **symptoms** of a disease, usually an incurable one.

Resistant Immune to or unaffected by. (See also **bacterial resistance.**)

Respiratory Refers to the body's breathing apparatus: the air passages extending from mouth and nostrils down through the throat and trachea to the **bronchi** and lungs.

Retrospective By hindsight: conclusions derived from past experience to estimate future results. Prospective means setting up observations or experiments ahead of time to study future events as they happen. Thus, a retrospective **clinical** trial may involve analyses of many case histories in a hospital's files while a prospective study records how patients respond to a **protocol** set up in advance.

Reversible Curable; capable of recovering from all signs of illness, injury, or disability. (See also **irreversible.**)

Rheumatic Having to do with rheumatism—sore, stiff, inflamed joints and muscles due to various causes, known and unknown.

Rheumatology A branch of medical science dealing with **rheumatic** diseases (such as rheumatoid arthritis and gout) or diseases of **connective tissue.**

Salicylates A class of **compounds** (of which aspirin is the best known) used to relieve pain, reduce **inflammation,** and lower body temperature.

Schizophrenia One of a group of **psychoses** in which the affected person undergoes personality changes marked by withdrawal and bizarre behavior. Hallucinations, delusions, and paranoia are not uncommon.

Screening Test A mass examination of a large group designed to detect a particular disease early enough to treat it with maximum effect.

Sebum A thick greasy **exudate;** a normal **secretion** of the sebaceous glands of skin and scalp.

Secondary Infection An **infection** that flares up in a tissue or organ made vulnerable by a prior infection. For example, **bacteria** may secondarily infect a fever blister originally caused by a **virus.**

Secretion The product of a gland or glands in the body. An external secretion (usually a complex mixture of organic chemicals) is produced by a nonendocrine gland and is ultimately extruded onto the body's surface; e.g., **sebum** is the secretion of a sebaceous gland; **mucus** is the secretion of **respiratory** or **gastrointestinal** glands; tears are the secretion of the lachrymal glands. An internal secretion, usually a **hormone,** is delivered directly into the bloodstream from its site of manufacture in one of the glands of the **endocrine system.**

Sedative A **drug** that exerts a calming or quieting effect on mental processes or nervous irritability. (See also **hypnotic, tranquilizer.**)

Sensitization Stimulation of the body's **immunological response** "memory" by a foreign substance, so that the next time the alien material makes contact—which may be even years later—**symptoms** of the **allergy** may appear.

Serum Factors In the serum (the liquid part of the blood) there are various types of **antibodies** that help the **white blood cells** to overwhelm infecting **microorganisms.** Serum factors may also be associated with certain diseases such as rheumatoid arthritis (see **rheumatology**) or thyroiditis.

Shotgun Remedy A medication combining two or more different therapeutic **drugs** in a single preparation, presumably based on the theory that if enough ingredients are used, one might work.

Side Effect The cloud inside the silver lining. Every **drug,** along with its desired **pharmacological** action, causes other gratuitous consequences, ranging from incidental to downright **toxic.** Because these dividends—usually unwelcome—may be dose-related, proper **chemotherapy** must specify the exact quantity of **drugs** that offers the best tradeoff between benefit to the patient, and the possibility of burden to the body.

Sign See **symptom.**

Sitz Bath Fundamental bliss: a warm bath, with or without added salts, in which a patient sits with hips and buttocks under water. *Sitz* means "seat" in German.

Smear A sample of blood, **mucus,** pus, or other material from the body spread on a glass slide for staining and examination under a microscope.

Sodium   One of the two chemical elements in table salt (the other is chlorine). In the body, sodium is one of the most important constituents of blood and of other body fluids. People with **congestive heart failure** or **hypertension** may be advised to reduce sodium in their diet.

Spasm   Involuntary contraction (clenching, tensing, or tightening up) of muscles.

Spectrum   Assortment, array. Originally described the range of wavelengths—the rainbow in the sky spanning the spectrum of visible colors. Now refers to any range or span or set of effects, such as a broad-spectrum **antibiotic,** which is effective against both **Gram-positive** and **Gram-negative bacteria** or a variety of disease **symptoms.**

Sphincter   A round muscle encircling an opening in the body; when it contracts, it is capable of closing the orifice.

Sputum   **Mucus,** sometimes mixed with pus, coughed up from the lungs and **bronchi.** Synonym: phlegm.

Steroids   A family of organic **compounds,** or their **analogues,** of which the **corticosteroid hormones** secreted by the **adrenal glands** are a subdivision. Steroids perform a vital function in the process of **metabolism.**

Subacute   Midway between **acute** and **chronic** in the course of a disease.

Suspension   A uniform mixture of insoluble fine particles in water or some other liquid. Liquid **antacids** are usually suspensions.

Sutures   Stitches, clamps, or staples applied by a surgeon to hold the edges of a wound together until they heal.

Sympathetic Nervous System   (Derived from sympathin, the old name for **adrenaline.**) A network of nerves that trigger certain involuntary or automatic bodily functions, such as constricting blood vessels, making hair stand on end, raising "gooseflesh" on the skin, widening the pupils, contracting most **sphincters,** and speeding up the heartbeat. These stimuli add up to the "startle reaction" by which the body mobilizes for "fight or flight" in the face of sudden danger or surprise. (See also **central nervous system, parasympathetic nervous system.**)

Symptom   What the patient complains of—from bad breath to palpitations to pain. A symptom is your body's signal to you that something is wrong (e.g., abdominal pain) and a clue to your doctor as to what its cause is likely to be. A **sign** is what your doctor finds on examination (e.g., tenderness of the abdomen). One sign or symptom is not a **syndrome,** but several signs and symptoms are.

Symptomatic Relief   The amelioration of **symptoms** of disease by such measures as the **administration** of medicine. For example, aspirin is commonly used for relief of pain, which is a symptom, rather than as treatment for the underlying cause of the pain.

Syndrome A set or constellation of **symptoms** or signs that together characterize or identify a specific disease or disorder.

Synergistic The whole being greater than the sum of its parts. That is, when two or more effects applied at the same time multiply rather than add up their consequences. Thus, two **drugs** taken together may act synergistically—their effect is more than just the sum of each used separately.

Systemic Referring to the body as a whole, rather than to **one** of its parts.

Therapeutic Equivalent A **drug** that can be substituted for another without loss of efficacy.

Therapy Any form of medical treatment.

Thrombosed Refers to a vein or artery being plugged or clogged with clotted blood. When the thrombus (or clot) breaks loose and travels to another organ it is called an embolus and results in an embolism.

Time-Release A form of medication in which the active **drug** is purportedly absorbed into the bloodstream gradually over an extended period. Actually, the release rate may be highly variable from person to person and dose to dose.

Tolerance The process by which the body adjusts to the effects of a **drug** and thus requires increased or more frequent dosages to achieve the desired effects. (See also **addicting, rebound effect**.)

Tone A steady state of "stretch" or tension in healthy muscles enabling them to be always ready to respond rapidly to stimuli. Certain diseases diminish this normal tonicity, rendering muscles **atonic**.

Topical Applied directly on the skin (or accessible **mucous membrane**) to treat a **lesion** at its local site, rather than administered systemically (i.e., throughout the body, by way of the bloodstream or digestive tract).

Tourniquet A cord, cloth, or something similar twisted around a wounded limb to stop blood loss. This old-time first-aid standby is now rarely recommended. Hand pressure or a pressure bandage is usually as effective, and far safer.

Toxic Poisonous: effect ranging from harmful to lethal, depending on the dose taken and the resistance of the individual. (See also **detoxify**.)

Tranquilizer A **drug** used to relieve anxiety and to calm. Major tranquilizers are used to treat **psychoses;** minor tranquilizers are used to relieve **symptoms** of anxiety and, sometimes, to relieve emotional stress associated with **organic disease.** Because it is less likely to produce drowsiness, a tranquilizer may be preferable to a **sedative,** particularly for daytime use.

Trimester The first, second, or third three-month period of the nine months of pregnancy.

Troche A pill or lozenge that is dissolved in the mouth.

Tumor An abnormal growth on or in the body, which serves no useful purpose. A tumor may be malignant (cancerous) or benign (noncancerous).

Urethra A narrow channel (shorter in women than in men) through which the bladder voids urine. When the urethra is narrowed, as may happen with recurrent infection, it may have to be surgically stretched (dilated) to restore outflow.

Urology A branch of surgery dealing with the urinary tract—kidneys, ureters, bladder, **urethra**—plus (in males) the prostate gland and genitals.

USP Refers to a **drug** compounded according to the *United States Pharmacopeia,* a semiofficial **pharmacological** directory of drug standards and specifications, issued every five years by a national committee of physicians, pharmacists, and academicians. (See also **NF**.)

Vaccine A specially formulated mix of a weakened or killed **infection**-causing **bacterium** or **virus** introduced into the body so that the body through its immune mechanism will develop **antibodies** against the same bacterium or virus. These antibodies serve as protection against infection with the naturally occurring bacterium or virus.

Vaporizer A device for adding moisture or humidity to the air of a room. A cool-mist model does this by atomizing water into microdroplets. An electrolytic vaporizer boils water to steam up the atmosphere. An ultrasonic model uses sound waves to create a mist.

Varicose Veins Abnormal veins that have become permanently stretched. There is an increased tendency for blood flow to slow down and for clots to form in these veins. Varicose veins usually occur in the legs and the anal region.

Vascular About the blood's delivery system—arteries, veins, **capillaries**.

Vasoconstrictor A chemical substance that narrows or shrinks the diameter of arteries and thereby reduces blood supply to an organ or tissue.

Vasomotor Concerning or affecting the mechanism by which the walls of blood vessels expand and contract to regulate blood flow, blood pressure, and body temperature.

Vector Anything that transmits **infection** from one **host** to another. Thus, a mosquito is the vector of malaria; a kiss (actually saliva) may be a vector of the common cold.

Virus This smallest of all **microorganisms** causes a variety of viral **infections,** from fever blisters and German measles to poliomyelitis. Some viruses are suspected of triggering certain cancers. A virus causes havoc by invading a cell, disrupting its internal functioning, and distorting its reproduction mechanism.

White Blood Cells Cells in the bloodstream that fight off **infection** by harmful **microorganisms.** One kind of white cell actually attacks **bacteria.** The other kind helps by making **antibodies.** Dead white cells and tissue, along with killed bacteria, collect as pus. (See also **serum factors**.)

PRODUCT INDEX

GENERAL INDEX

Abbott Laboratories, 132, 273
Acesulfame K, 130, 137–38
Acetaminophen, 7, 10–11, 12, 13, 15–17, 26; comparison to other analgesics, 13–14
Acid-base balance of the body, 50
Acid foods, 46–47
Acid neutralizing capacity, 48–49
Acidophilus milk, 64
"Acid rebound," 50
Acne, 151–58; OTC remedies for, 152–53; prescription drugs for, 153–56; self-treatment of, 156–58; understanding of, 151–52
Aconite, 256
Acquired immune deficiency syndrome, see AIDS
Active ingredients in drugs, 2–3
Acute gastroenteritis, see Diarrhea
Additives, food, 220
Adolescents: calcium needs of, 202
Adrenal glands, 107
Advertising of drugs, 271–72
Africans, central, AIDS among, 236, 240–41
Age and hypertension, 109
AIDS, 231–41, 242; fear of, 231–32; safety of blood supply and, 242, 242–43, 249; testing for, 233–34, 242–43, 249; transmission of, 231, 232, 234–38; ways it is not transmitted, 239–41
AIDS-related complex (ARC), 233
Air-conditioning, 36
Albuterol, 41
Alcohol, 46, 81, 92, 111, 201–2, 209; birth defects and, 218–19; insomnia and, 75, 77–78
Alcoholics, acetaminophen and, 11
Alkylamines, 31–32
Allergic rhinitis, see Hay fever
Allergies, 30–44, 72, 103, 163, 216; antihistamines for, 21–22, 31–32, 43–44; asthma and, 40–41; cause of, 30–31; decongestants for, 32–34; food, and intolerances, 30, 41–43; to mercury, 193–94, 196; professional help for, 35–37; recommendations,

43–44; self-treatment with OTCs, 31–35; shotgun remedies for, 34–35; shots for, 37–40, 44; see also specific allergies
Aloe, 163
"Alternative Dietary Practices and Nutritional Abuses in Pregnancy," 219
Aluminum, 51–52, 54, 55, 202
Aluminum hydroxide, 51–52
Alzheimer's disease, 52
Amebic dysentery, 59
American Dental Association, 183, 192
American Heart Association, 85, 105; diet of, 88, 89, 93, 95, 97
American Medical Association, 245; Council on Scientific Affairs, 37, 137
American Pharmaceutical Association, 13, 17
American Red Cross, 243, 245, 248
Amsterdam (Netherlands) Municipal Health Service, 238
Analgesics, 7–17, 114; acetaminophen, see Acetaminophen; aspirin, see Aspirin; for cold-related pain, 26; comparing pain relief of, 13–14; ibuprofen, see Ibuprofen; menstrual pain and, 11–12, 14–15; selecting, 15–17; with several ingredients, 12–13
Anal hygiene, 70, 71
Anal intercourse, 234, 235
Anemia, iron-deficiency, 9, 146, 248
Anesthetics, 72
Angina, 256; aspirin and, 8
Antacids, 45–58, 60, 61, 202; in aspirin, 9–12; effectiveness of, 48–49; heartburn prevention and relief, 46–47; ingredients, 49–53; recommendations, 54–55; for ulcers and gastritis, 47–48
Antibiotics, 70, 153–54, 190, 216
Anticoagulants, 8, 16, 102
Antidepressants, 61
Antihistamines: for allergies, 21, 31–34, 36, 43–44; in cold remedies, 20–21; in sleep aids, 78
Anti-inflammatories, 8, 11